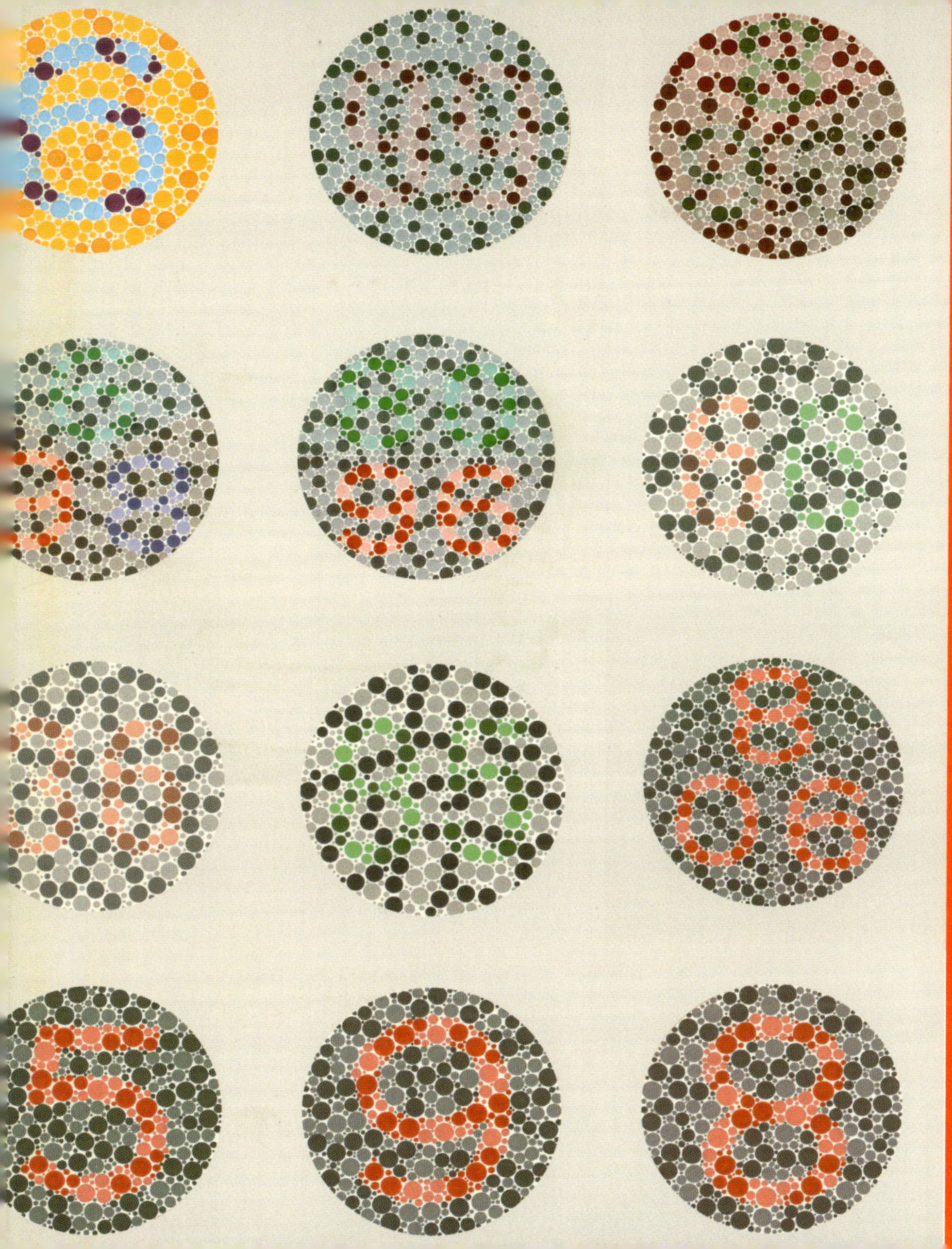

COLOR
VISION TEST
PLATES

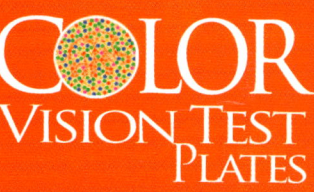

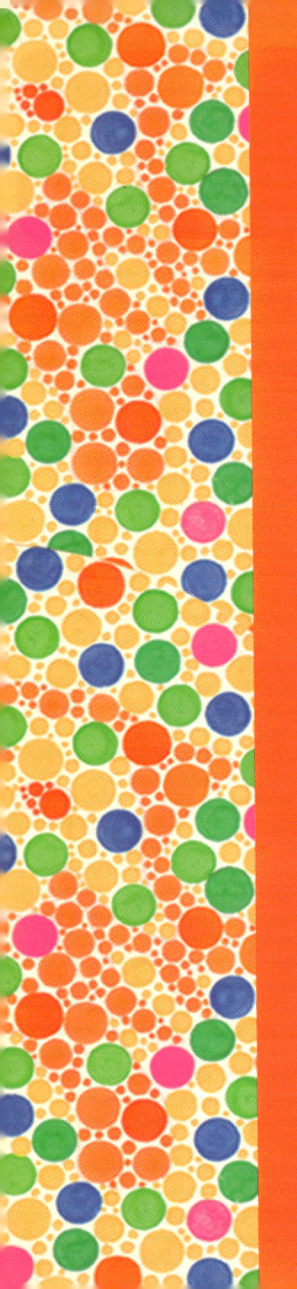

Project Editor: Zuo Wei

Book Designer: Zhao Jing-jin

Cover Designer: Zhao Jing-jin

Typesetter: Wei Hong-bo

Kezhang Wang   Xinyu Wang

COLOR
VISION TEST
PLATES

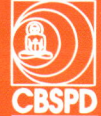

CBSPD

CBS Publishers & Distributors Pvt Ltd

New Delhi • Bengaluru • Chennai • Kochi • Kolkata • Lucknow • Mumbai

Gujarat • Hyderabad • Jharkhand • Nagpur • Patna • Pune • Uttarakhand

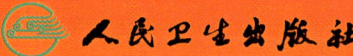

人民卫生出版社

PMPH   PEOPLE'S MEDICAL PUBLISHING HOUSE

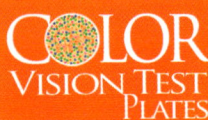

Book Title: Color Vision Test Plates 色觉检查图

ISBN: 978-93-86827-70-8

CBS Edition: 2019, **2026**

This edition has been published by CBS Publishers & Distributors under arrangement with People's Medical Publishing House

First published: 2008

PMPH ISBN: 978-7-117-09176-3/R·9177

Not for sale outside India, Pakistan, Nepal, Bhutan and Sri Lanka.

Cataloguing in Publication Data: A catalog record for this book is available from the CIP-Database China.

Published by **Satish Kumar Jain** and produced by **Varun Jain** for

CBS Publishers & Distributors Pvt Ltd

4819/XI Prahlad Street, 24 Ansari Road, Daryaganj, New Delhi 110 002, India
Ph: 011-23289259, 23266838   Website: www.cbspd.com   e-mail: delhi@cbspd.com
Corporate Office: 204 FIE, Industrial Area, Patparganj, Delhi 110 092, India
Ph: 011-49344934   Fax: 011-49344935   e-mail: publishing@cbspd.com; publicity@cbspd.com

Branches

- **Bengaluru:** Seema House 2975, 17th Cross, K.R. Road, Banasankari 2nd Stage, Bengaluru 560 070, Karnataka, India
  Ph: +91-80-26771678/79   Fax: +91-80-26771680   e-mail: bangalore@cbspd.com
- **Chennai:** 18/8B, Subbarayan Street, Shenoy Nagar, Chennai 600 030, Tamil Nadu, India
  Ph: +91-44-42032115, 26681266   e-mail: chennai@cbspd.com
- **Kochi:** 42/1325, 1326, Power House Road, Opposite KSEB, Power House, Ernakulum 682018, Kochi, Kerala, India
  Ph: +91-484-4059061–65   Fax: +91-484-4059065   e-mail: kochi@cbspd.com
- **Kolkata:** 147, Hind Ceramics Compound, 1st Floor, Nilgunj Road, Belghoria, Kolkata 700056, West Bengal, India
  Ph: +91-33-25330055/56   e-mail: kolkata@cbspd.com
- **Lucknow:** Basement, Khushuma Complex, 7 Meerabai Marg (behind Jawahar Bhawan), Lucknow 226001, UP, India
  Ph: +91-522-4000032   e-mail: tiwari.lucknow@cbspd.com
- **Mumbai:** PWD Shed, Gala No. 25/26, Ramchandra Bhatt Marg, Next JJ Hospital, Gate No. 2, Opp. Union Bank of India, Noorbaug, Mumbai 400009, Maharashtra, India
  Ph: +91-22-66661880/89   e-mail: mumbai@cbspd.com

Representatives

• **Gujarat**	0-9879558667	• **Hyderabad**	0-9885175004	• **Jharkhand**	0-9811541605
• **Nagpur**	0-8692091830	• **Patna**	0-9334159340	• **Pune**	0-9664372571
• **Uttarakhand**	0-9716462459				

Printed at Sri Print and Sales, Delhi, India

PREFACE

PROLEGOMENON

PRACTICAL MANUAL FOR COLOR VISION TEST PLATES

1. Color vision anomaly in clinic
2. Types of color blindness
3. Test for color vision defects
4. Basis of plates devising and how to use this book
5. Attention to use this book
6. Direction Chart For the Plates

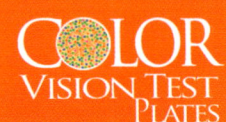

PREFACE

As a kind of medical examination, color vision test plays an important role in employment. Through ten years of hard work, according to the pseudo-isochromatic theory, Professor Kezhang Wang drew a lot of rich, comprehensive and normative color vision plates (testified by the automatic color difference meter) based on the theory of color vision and the theory of complementary color. These plates can be realistically printed easily. Some improvements had been made in this book on the basis of the advanced information in this field. This book can be used in testing of red, green, yellow and blue (violet) color vision, and classify the red, green and blue (violet) color weakness into three degrees, i.e. strong, medium, mild degree. Therefore, the color vision test could be achieved qualitatively and quasi-quantitatively. It has been proved in clinic that this book is a very convenient, highly sensitive, credible and useful tool. Above is the short introduction to the book before publication. Sincerely wish the experts in ophthalmology make some recommendations to this book selflessly. Any advice and suggestion is highly appreciated.

Jun Yang

Write in Beijing, on January 1992

PROLEGOMENON

Visual function test is composed of eyesight, visual field, color vision and electrophysiological examination, in which the eyesight and color vision test are common and necessary in medical examination. Using the color vision plates is the most convenient, fast and accurate method in clinic.

Color vision is the capacity of a person to recognize objects based on the wavelengths (or frequencies) of the light they reflect or emit. Electromagnetic of certain wavelength range could stimulate the visual organ of mankind and then the vision system process the information of stimulation so that the color vision is produced. Any change of the components in the vision system would make the change of the eyesight or color vision.

The color vision anomaly is mostly congenital, but sometimes it could also be made by some diseases and traumatisms and this kind of anomaly is called acquired color blindness. The congenital patients often cannot detect their diseases by themselves if not by the medical examination, who just think their color vision are the same as the normal's, but in fact the colors they perceived are different from the normal. Normal people can easily see a red flag in blue sky, but for patient with red-green color blindness that is difficult. According to the current researches, there are about 4%-5% of color anomaly person and more percentages of color weakness patients in the world. The congenital color vision anomaly comes into being mostly by descendiblity.

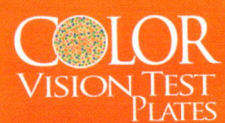

Our world is more and more colorful with the development of scientific technology. Three-dimensional traffic network from the air to earth is complicated; we often control it through indicative lights of different colors. The red and green traffic light is familiar to us. Compared to normal people, it is more difficult for color vision anomaly especially the patients with color blindness to distinguish the signals who can just distinguish them through the position of lights or follow the front cars. It is dangerous because they often make mistakes.

A train collision occurred in Sweden in 1875 because the train driver was color blindness who made mistakes for the traffic signals. In 1876, Sweden made the rule that employees of railway and sailors must pass the test for color blindness. Then Germany, Austria and Japan set up this rule as well. The color vision test is part of routine medical examination now.

Test of color vision is very important for selecting a person of talent, especially the jobs which require high standard on the color perception. The color deficiency patients can also find their own jobs basis on their special anomaly.

We can't do the color vision test by one kind of instruments, neither too complicated nor too simple. There are several types of color vision test instruments, including Nagel anomaloscope, FM-100 hue test, and color vision test plates which is most convenient in clinic.

There is a new challenge for the research of color vision test during the modern technology developing. Basis on the condition of daedal lighting instruments, color vision distinguishing under special circumstance, and reading of computer figure, which make the visual research developing, we should lucubrate the visual function of human and apply it into our work and daily life. Of course, people should understand their own visual and color vision function. In a word, the color vision test is essential for us.

This book was compiled based on the theory of color vision and law of complementary colors in Chromatics and the theory of pseudo-isochromatic. According to the CIE chromaticity diagram and the 1975 standard of light signal color, the primary colors, red, green, yellow and blue (violet) were chosen among the chromaticity arrange of the CIE chromaticity diagram. The coordinate color and the demitints with different contents of red or green color, which were quantificationally measured by the PC-P II automatic color difference meter, were tested, used, amended a few times and finally confirmed.

This book has been published 5 times since 1993 in China. According to different situations of clinic, the plates of this book were amended, especially supplemented some new plates which were made by computer. Currently, there are 66 plates in this book, which can be divided into three parts. The first part, number group, there are 38 plates, which are plates of test for red, green, blue (violet) and yellow blindness and weakness, which divide color weakness into 3 degree: strong, medium and mild degree for red, green and blue (violet) color weakness. The second part, Latin letter group, which fits to the patient with quickly check or re-check. The third part, animal pictures group, there are 15 plates, which fit children and illiterates. The plate 35, plate 36, plate 37, plate 38, and plate 66 are tests for tiredness of color vision and latent color blindness.

This book has been tested for more than 10,000 times in clinic, and it was proved that the book with high sensitivity could take qualitative and quasi-quantitative tests to color vision anomaly patients.

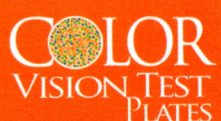

Thanks for Tianshui Science Technology Bureau, and thanks for Professor Jun Yang, Professor Ziping Yu and Professor Yanhua Wang who are famous ophthalmologists in China took a appraisal on this book on December 1989.

This book supported by Gansu Provincial Sci.&Tech. Department, Tianshui Science Technology Bureau and Tianshui First People's Hospital. Thanks for Professor Jun Yang, Professor Ziping Yu, Professor Yanhua Wang, Professor Xiaolou Zhang, Professor Yuanxiu Lao, Professor Lingzhi Zhang, Professor of Medicine Xuemin Zhu, Professor of Medicine Benbao Zou, Professor of Medicine Ruwen He, Professor of Medicine Kehui Shen, Engineer Mingming Sheng, Associate Professor of Medicine Shaotuo Cai. Thanks for the help of Associate Professor of Medicine Jiaqi Lei.

Sincerely wish the experts in ophthalmology and users make some recommendations to this book.

Kezhang Wang

2001.02

Practical Manual
for Color Vision Test Plates

1. Color vision anomaly in clinic

People with abnormal color vision are called color vision anomaly, or color vision defect. According to the color blindness statistic in China from 1932 to 1957, male patients are about 5.14% to the total population, and female patients are about 0.73%. Male patients are more about 7 times than that of female. In Japan, male patients are about 4%-5% of the total population; female patients are about 0.5%. And in Europe, male patients are about 8% to the total population; female patients are about 0.4%. The numbers of every kind of color blindness are different. According to the methods for classifying color blindness of Von Kries, the types of color blindness classified by Wright shows on the following table:

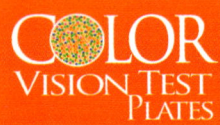

The types and percentage of color vision anomaly

Type		Percentage
Anomalous trichromat	Red color vision anomaly Green color vision anomaly	1.0 4.6
Anomalous dichromat	Red blindness Green blindness	1.2 1.4
Monochromat		0.003
Total		8.2

Based on this table, we can see that the patients with green color anomaly are more than that with red. The monochromat patients have been founded rarely.

Color vision defect can be grouped as color vision weakness and color blindness. Patient with color weakness, whose ability of recognizing colors has degenerated or lacked, can read the colors in the condition of bright light, deep hue, extensive visual angle, and need more time, otherwise, the patient can't recognize color as normal person. The patients with color weakness can be rated as different degrees and their eyesights are independent of the color weakness degrees. Some of weakness patients are better than color blindness, and they may remain some parts of color identifying ability. Some of them whose ability of recognizing color is not as good as normal person, can't recognize color that is in lower saturation and chromatism. Some patients' symptoms are just between the above two kinds of weakness. Therefore, the experts categorized the color weakness into three types earlier which are degree A, degree B, degree C to show the severity of the weakness. And there are three degrees too in this book that are strong, medium, and mild degrees.

Color blindness means person can't recognize different colors, i.e. lacking the ability of recognizing colors. Patients with red or green blindness are more common in clinic and yellow or blue blindness patients are fewer. Total color blindness patients can't distinguish colors completely, who can only recognize the shape, bright and dark of objects, and sense red and green colors darker, yellow and blue brighter, and also have photophobia, frequent nictation and bad eyesight which will be more serious in blazing light and be better in weak light. The central scotoma will be found in perimetry and the peripheral visual field is natural. The central scotoma which can cause intermittent nystagmus will be founded when doing visual field examination. To the ability of adaptation for scotopic vision, the one with total color blindness is better than normal person. The normal person usually needs 5-10 minutes to adapt the dark condition, but the total color blindness patient only needs 1-2 minutes. To the total color blindness, the brightest area in spectrum is the band of green color, which is different to the normal person whose brightest area is band of yellow generally but is green band only in the condition of lacking light. Therefore, the sense of total blindness is the same as the sense of the normal eye when they stayed in dark room for a long time.

Patients with red, green color blindness or weakness are the most common in color vision anomaly who can distinguish yellow and blue color when the two colors' aberrations are obvious enough. But they read red or green color as grey or brown which is the same as the middle color mixed by red and green to normal person.

The patient with red blindness whose ability of recognizing green color is abnormal too, read the red band of the spectrum as grey which looks shortened, and the brightest band of spectrum is yellow-green band.

The patient with green blindness, who can't recognize red and green colors but with any

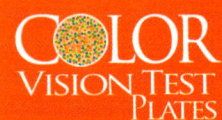

shortness of red color band, will read the spectrum band of green color as neutral band, and the brightest band of the spectrum is orange color.

Patients with yellow, blue (violet) color blindness are rare in clinic; they can't recognize the band of yellow and blue (violet) colors; they may read the band of yellow and blue (violet) colors as neutral band, and the brightest band of the spectrum is the yellow one.

2. Types of color blindness

Color blindness occurs both as a congenital and as an acquired defect. Congenital color blindness is known as Daltonism, after the English physicist Dalton, who was color-blind himself, and who was the first to describe the defect accurately. Color blindness occurs, as most of in the intermarriage family, that the defect is in many cases inherited, being transmitted as sex-linked recessives, that is, remaining latent in the female and becoming manifest only in the male offspring. That means male color blindness whose daughter's son will be transmitted. Because female is latent carrier that female color blindness is less than male color blindness in the clinic.

Acquired color vision defects can be caused by three kinds of reasons: refraction structures changes, psychiatric disorders and visual pathway damages.

The diseases which result in acquired color blindness are listed as follow:

Disease	*color vision defect*
Congenital jaundice	Extreme deuteranomaly

Albinism	Extreme deuteranomaly
Peripheral pigmentary dystrophy	Deuteranopia, blue-yellow and red-green defects
Central pigmentary dystrophy	Red-green and blue-yellow
Albipunctate dystrophy	Blue-yellow
Choroideremia	Blue-yellow
Sorsby's dystrophy	Red-green
Choroidal sclerosis	Blue-yellow and red-green
Fuchs's gyrate atrophy	Red-green
Vogt-Spielmeyer's disease	Red-green
Juvenile macular degeneration	Red-green
Senile macular degeneration	Blue-yellow
Grönblad-Strandberg syndrome	Blue-yellow
Cystic macular degeneration	Congenital:deuteranopia
Retinoschisis	Blue-yellow
Malignant myopia	Blue-yellow, red-green
Siderosis	Blue-yellow
Chorioretinitis	Blue-yellow
Central serous retinopathy	Blue-yellow
Hypertensive retinopathy	Blue-yellow
Diabetic retinopathy	Blue-yellow
Retinal vascular occlusions	Blue-yellow
Choroidal malignant melanoma	Blue-yellow
Glaucoma	Blue-yellow
Drusen of the optic disc	Red-green, blue-yellow
Retrobulbar neuritis	Red-green

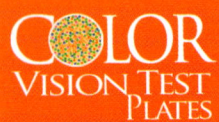

| | | Chiasmal lesions | | Red-green |
| | | Alcohol-nicotine intoxication | | Red-green |

The ability of color distinguishing will degenerate when the human gets older.

Current classification of color blindness is shown in the following chart :

COLOR-VISION	Trichromat	Normal	
		Anomalous	Protanomaly
			Deuteranomaly
			Tritanomaly
	Dichromat	Protanopia (Red blindness)	
		Deuteranopia (Green blindness)	
		Acyanopsia (Blue-violet blindness)	
	Monochromat (Total color blindness)		

The plates in this book classified weakness of red, green and blue (violet) color into three categories as high-degree (a little ability of recognizing color vision, nearest color blindness), middle-degree (little more ability of recognizing color vision) and low-degree (more ability of recognizing color vision). The book mainly uses classification of the weakness of red and green color, because blue (violet) color vision anomaly is very rare.

In addition, there are also tiredness of color vision and latent color blindness in clinic. The tiredness of color vision is that human beings can quickly recognize color at the beginning of the test, but patient can't do it or deny preliminary results when the test is longer or the colors are complex, high contrast or dazzling. And patient can recognize color again when he get rest. The latent color blindness is that a person has color receptors in retina, but behaves just like those with red or green color blindness when recognizing color. The patient need more time to discriminate color when taking color vision test, especially those plates with little difference. That means their eyes have color receptors, but they can't recognize color like normal. They have less sensitivity of the color and need more time than normal person to recognize the right color. Patients of this kind have less chemic sensitive substance in retina.

3. Test for color vision defects

Most of color defects patients are congenital, who thinks that they are normal person, because they never have experience of recognizing colors correctly. For example, the patient with red or green color blindness can recognize color by his way when the red or green color is shown obviously. Therefore, the color blindness only can be found when they take a test of color vision.

Long time ago, people found that color blindness test was very important. In 1875, a train crashed in Sweden, Holmgren who was physiologist, found the driver was color blind, and he saw signal lamp in a wrong way. That's why train crash was happened. In 1876, Sweden made the rule that employees of railway and sailor must pass the test for color blindness. Then Germany, Austria and Japan set up this rule as well. The color vision test is a part of routine medical examination now.

Currently, there are too many ways for color blindness test, for example, the color mixed test, Holmgren's color clew, the color pencil record and color light test. But usually the clinics use the plates of color blindness test.

The first plate of color blindness test was devised by Stilling, and then Ishihara made some

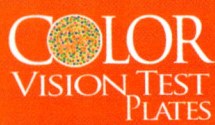

changes based on Stilling's. In 1936, charts of the color blindness test made by Крдс Нагел-Рабкин were used into clinics which were similar with that of Stilling. Color vision test is very important in some special fields, such as transportation, arts, physic, chemistry, air, navy, reconnaissance, geology, and military in which normal ability of recognizing color is needed.

4. Basis of plates devising and how to use this book

According to the theory of color vision, we should choose the red-green or yellow-blue (violet) colors for primary colors when we do test for color vision. In the chromatics, red-green or yellow-blue (purple) are complementary colors with each other. According to the pseudo-isochromatic theory, the integrated plates of color vision test were devised with mixture of colors that are based on that two pairs of complementary colors.

Red-green or yellow-blue (violet) can make a series of colors when they are mixed with each other. For example, in the series of red-green color, the red and green color which represent at the beginning and end of series, then turn to mixture color that is not red and not green which represent grey color which is neutral color on the middle line. That grey color occurred, which is grey-black with certain brightness but no multicolor, reflecting no homochromy color when two equal quantities complementary colors can completely absorbed the spectrum wavelengths each other. This is the same as color blindness patient who only can distinguish color brightness but can't recognize red or green color itself. Therefore, according to pseudo-isochromatic theory, we can devise plates of the color blindness test, which primary colors is red, green, blue (violet) and yellow, and then match color is the grey color which is neutral color of the series of complementary colors. Then according to pseudo-isochromatic theory, we can devise plates of test for color weakness with strong degree, medium degree and mild degree, which primary colors are red, green, blue (violet) and yellow, and match colors are middle colors which contain primary colors with different proportion and saturation. Using color difference meter to measure match colors of color weakness plates which are three middle colors selected from two series of complementary colors of red-green or yellow-blue (violet).

The method of testing abnormal color vision in this book is that the man who can't recognize the plates made by primaries colors which is red, green, blue (violet) and yellow, and match color which is neutral grey color (i.e. person has no perception of certain color), is what kind of color blindness is. According to tester's result, the patient who is red, green or blue (violet) color weakness, is rated as strong degree, medium degree or mild degree by the plates which are composed of primaries and middle colors which contain different hues. Most of color weakness patients are weak in red and green color in the clinic; therefore, main classification of color vision weakness in this book is the weakness of red and green color. We can take qualitative and quantitative tests to find red blindness, green blindness, red blindness together with green weakness, green blindness with red weakness, red weakness, green weakness, blue (violet) blindness, blue (violet) weakness, yellow blindness, and yellow weakness.

There are 66 plates for test, which includes three parts in this book.

First part, number group, there are 38 plates, which is the main part. There are plates of test for red, green, blue (violet) and yellow blindness, which can rate color weakness degree into strong, medium and mild degree for red, green and blue (violet) weakness. Patients with strong degree color weakness can recognize color blindness plates but can't recognize any

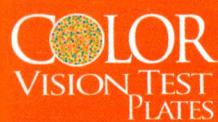

color weakness plates; patients with medium degree color weakness can recognize color blindness plates and strong degree color weakness plates but can't recognize medium degree color weakness plates; patients with mild degree color weakness can recognize color blindness plates and strong and medium degree color weakness plates but can't recognize mild degree color weakness plates. Normal person can distinguish any plates. The person who has high sensitivity of color vision can quickly recognize any plates. This proved test evidence for the job that needs high ability for distinguishing color. In physical examination, the tester should pick three plates from chart 2 to chart 8 and the normal person can read them all. If there were any problem, one need do more tests. Because this occurs only in few people, it could save time and avoid mistake this way.

Second part, Latin letter group, there are only 13 plates which patterns are easy and special, they fit to the patients who want to check quickly and re-check.

Third part, animal group, there are 15 plates which are novel and interesting and may use in children and illiterates.

The detail of how to use each plate shows on the plate manual (see section 3). The plate 35, plate 36, plate 37, plate 38, and plate 66 which are tests for tiredness of color vision and latent color blindness. These patients look like those with color weakness, but they are different. The plates are devised in contrary colors which are contrast and bright. Persons with normal color vision also feel dazzling when they see these plates, but they still can recognize correct colors when they distinguish carefully. However, patients with the tiredness of color vision can read at the beginning, and then will deny it when they continue looking at the plate. After a while, they can read again. Patients with latent color blindness can't read the plate immediately but they can recognize it after reading the plate again and again. Patient with red-green blindness or red-green weakness may read it, because red-green blindness can track the shade (bright and dark) on the plate, and red-green weakness can distinguish bright and dark, and has a little ability of distinguishing color. Therefore, these plates can't apply for test red-green blindness and red-green weakness.

5. Attention to use this book

1. The plates should be used under the bright daylight (not direct sunlight), or under the daylight lamp (not best effect).

2. The plates should be held at a distance of 40-80cm from the person being examined and the tester should teach correct reading method first, then do the test, and make diagnose (not more than 5 second for per plate).

3. According to illumination of plates, the tester can diagnose a testee is normal or abnormal, and which type and degree the abnormal person is. If not sure, the tester should repeat the test and compare with the former result. The plates for testing red, green blindness and weakness include united small pictures and single big pictures. Doctor can use two kinds of these plates to do test and compare the results on the basis of the single big pictures (see plates illumination).

4. No direct sunlight is allowed on the plate surface, the plates should be closed after being used in order to avoiding any color fading. When reading it, one should avoid wetting the plate surface. Both tester and testee should avoid touching the plates by finger, but a stick can be used instead if directions needed.

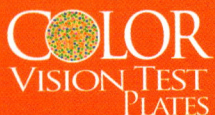

1.Arabic number group

Plate number	Normal	Color vision anomaly		Annotation
		Type	Result	
1	6		6	demonstration
2	99	Red-green color vision anomaly	0	Normal person also can read 0, abnormal person can only read 0
3	9 8 6	Red-green color blindness, strong degree of color weakness	Can't read it	Generally distinguish the red-green color blindness and red-green color weakness
		Medium degree color weakness	8	
		Mild degree color weakness	8 9	
4	9 6 8	Red-green color vision anomaly	8	Primary distinguish the red, green, blue(violet) color vision anomaly
		Red color vision anomaly	6 8	
		Green color vision anomaly	9 8	
		Blue(violet) color vision anomaly	6 9	
5	80 96	Red-green color vision anomaly	Can't read it	Distinguish red, green color vision anomaly
		Red color vision anomaly	80	
		Green color vision anomaly	96	
6	66	Red-green color blindness	Can't read it	Distinguish red-green color blindness
7	36	Red color blindness	Can't read it	Distinguish red color blindness
8	85	Green color blindness	Can't read it	Distinguish green color blindness
9	9 8 6	Red color blindness	Can't read it	The general plate for red color blindness

continued

Plate number	Normal	Color vision anomaly		Annotation
		Type	Result	
10	5	Red color blindness	Can't read it	Person who can't read two of three plates, is with red color blindness. Person who can read at least two plates, continue read the below plates for weakness
11	9	Red color blindness	Can't read it	
12	8	Red color blindness	Can't read it	
13	8 6 9	Green color blindness	Can't read it	The general plate for green color blindness
14	5	Green color blindness	Can't read it	Person who can't read two of three plates, is with green color blindness. Person who can read at least two plates, continue read the below plates for weakness
15	8	Green color blindness	Can't read it	
16	6	Green color blindness	Can't read it	
17	3 8 5	Red color weakness	Can't read it or can read partially	The general plate for red color weakness
18	3	Strong degree of red color weakness	Can't read it	These plates can rate the red weakness into strong, medium and mild degree
19	5	Medium degree of red color weakness	Can't read it	
20	8	Mild degree of red color weakness	Can't read it	
21	5 6 2	Green color weakness	Can't read it or can read partially	The general plate for green color weakness
22	8	Strong degree of green color weakness	Can't read it	These plates can be used to discriminate the green weakness into strong, medium and mild degree
23	9	Medium degree of green color weakness	Can't read it	
24	5	Mild degree of green color weakness	Can't read it	
25	83	Violet color blindness	Can't read it	Distinguish violet color blindness
26	6	Blue (violet) color blindness	Can't read it	The plate for blue(violet) color blindness

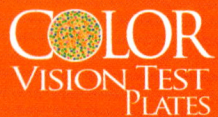

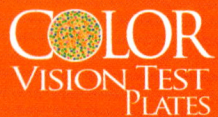 COLOR VISION TEST PLATES

continued

Plate number	Normal	Color vision anomaly		Annotation
		Type	Result	
27	3	Strong degree of blue (violet) color weakness	Can't read it	These plates can be used to discriminate the blue (violet) weakness into strong, medium and mild degree
28	5	Medium degree of blue (violet) color weakness	Can't read it	
29	8	Mild degree of blue (violet) color weakness	Can't read it	
30	56	Yellow blindness	Read it as 3	Distinguish yellow blindness
31	6	Yellow blindness	Can't read it	Distinguish yellow blindness
32	2	Strong degree of yellow color weakness	Can't read it	Distinguish yellow blindness
33	4	Medium degree of yellow color weakness	Can't read it	
34	9	Mild degree of yellow color weakness	Can't read it	
35	2	Tiredness of color vision	Can read it at beginning, then deny it later	Distinguish the tiredness of color vision and latent color blindness
		Latent color blindness	Can't read it at beginning, then maybe can read it later	
36	10	Tiredness of color vision	Can read it at beginning, then deny it later	Distinguish the tiredness of color vision and latent color blindness
		Latent color blindness	Can't read it at beginning, then maybe can read it later	
37	5	Tiredness of color vision	Can read it at beginning, then deny it later	Distinguish the tiredness of color vision and latent color blindness
		Latent color blindness	Can't read it at beginning, then maybe can read it later	
38	3	Tiredness of color vision	Can read it at beginning, then deny it later	Distinguish the tiredness of color vision and latent color blindness
		Latent color blindness	Can't read it at beginning, then maybe can read it later	

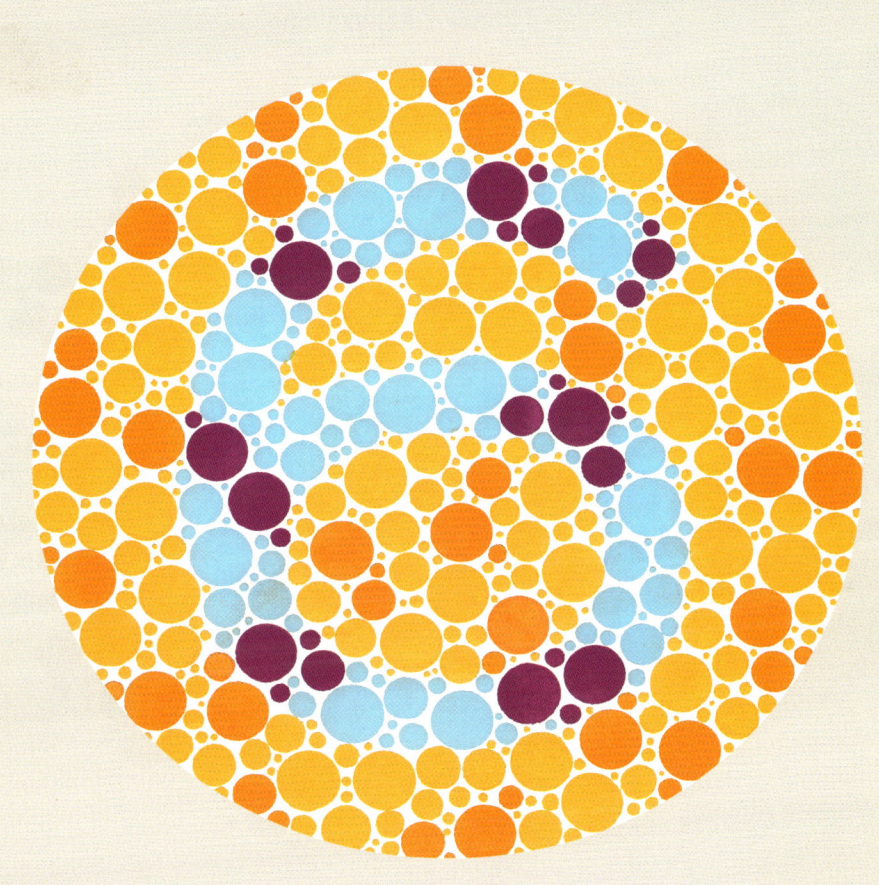

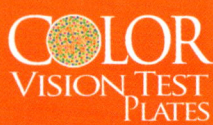

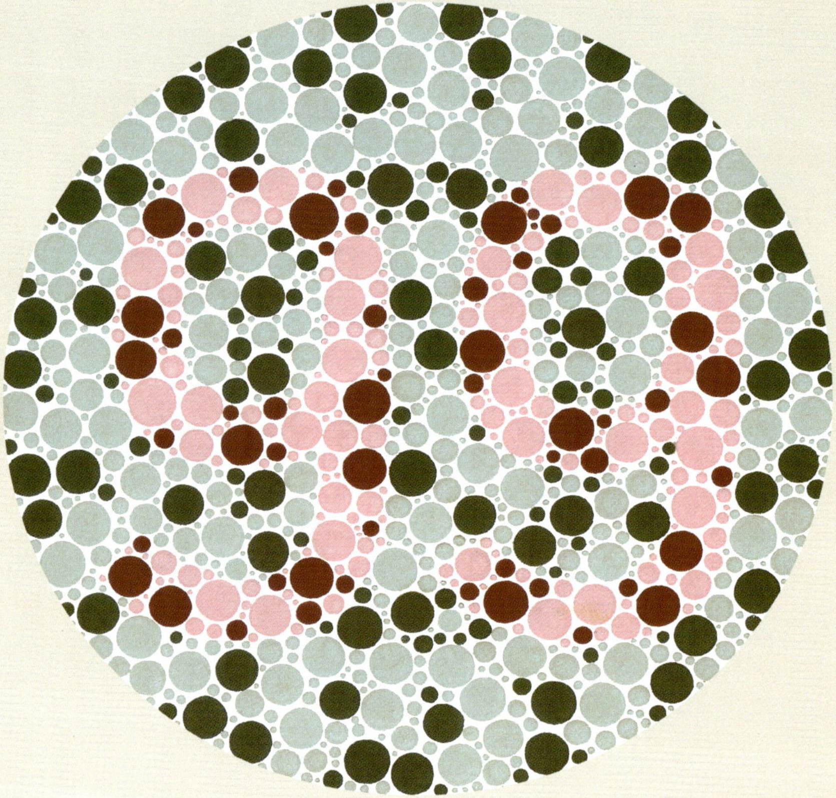

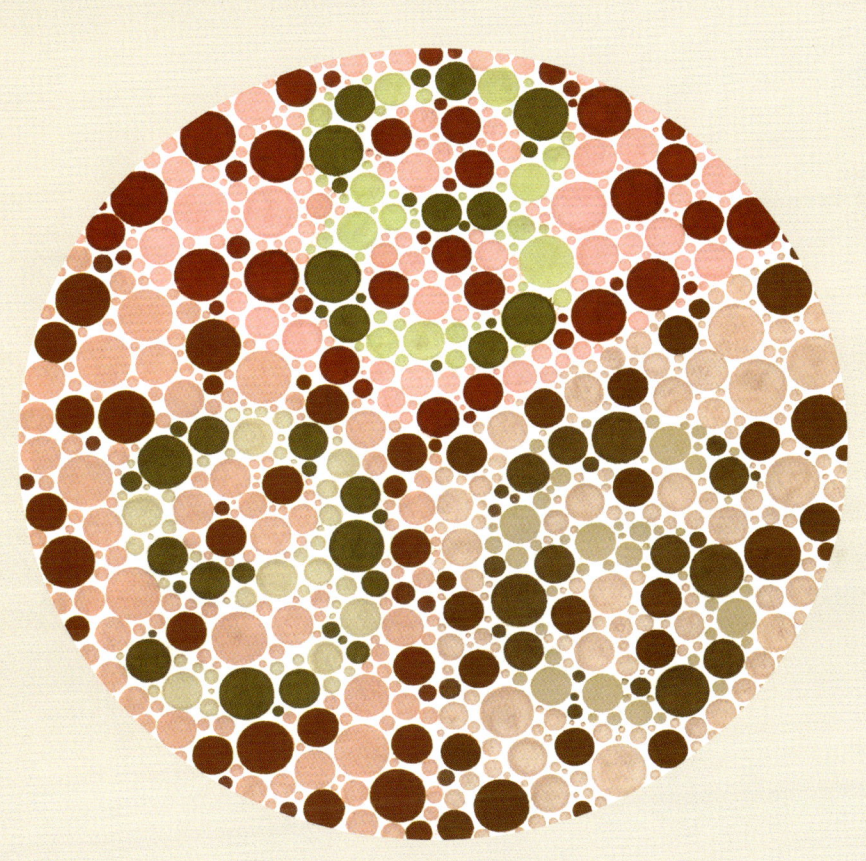

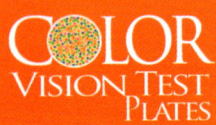

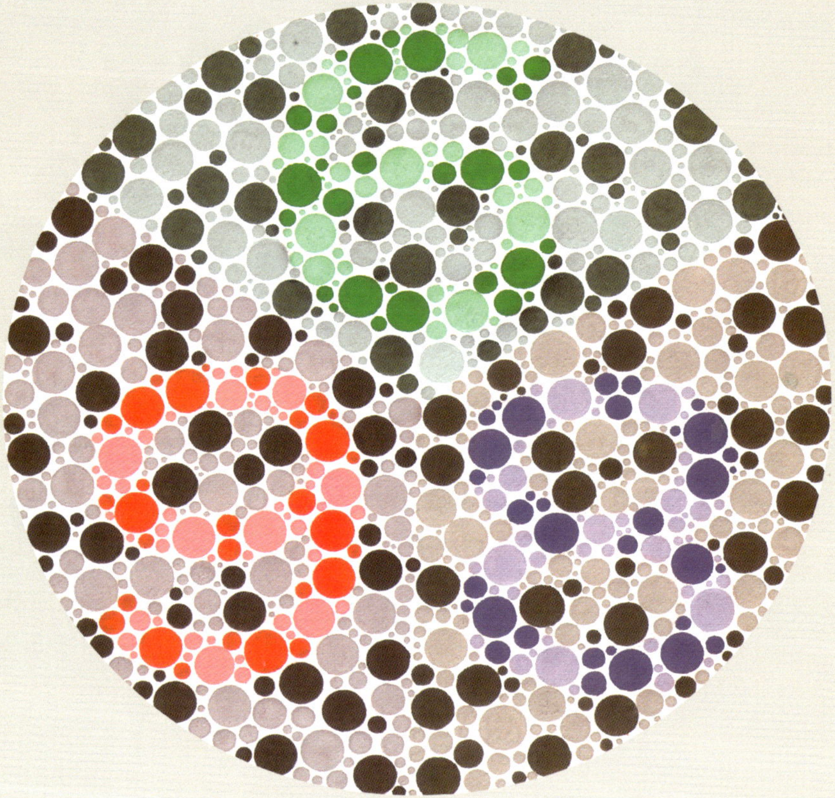

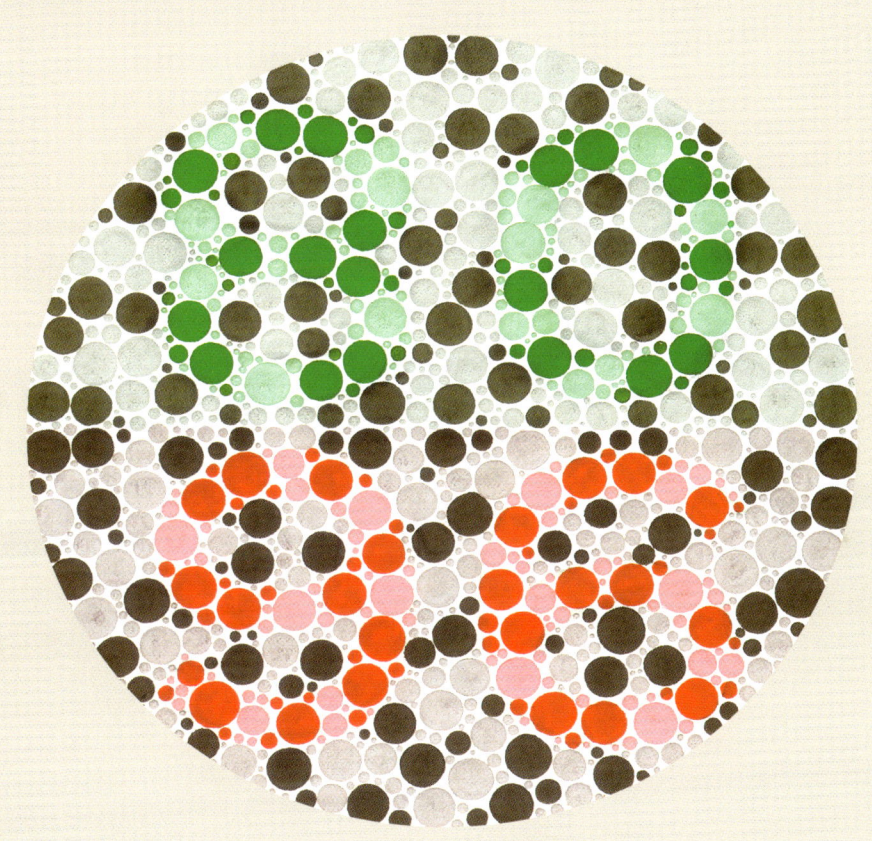

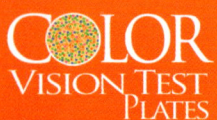

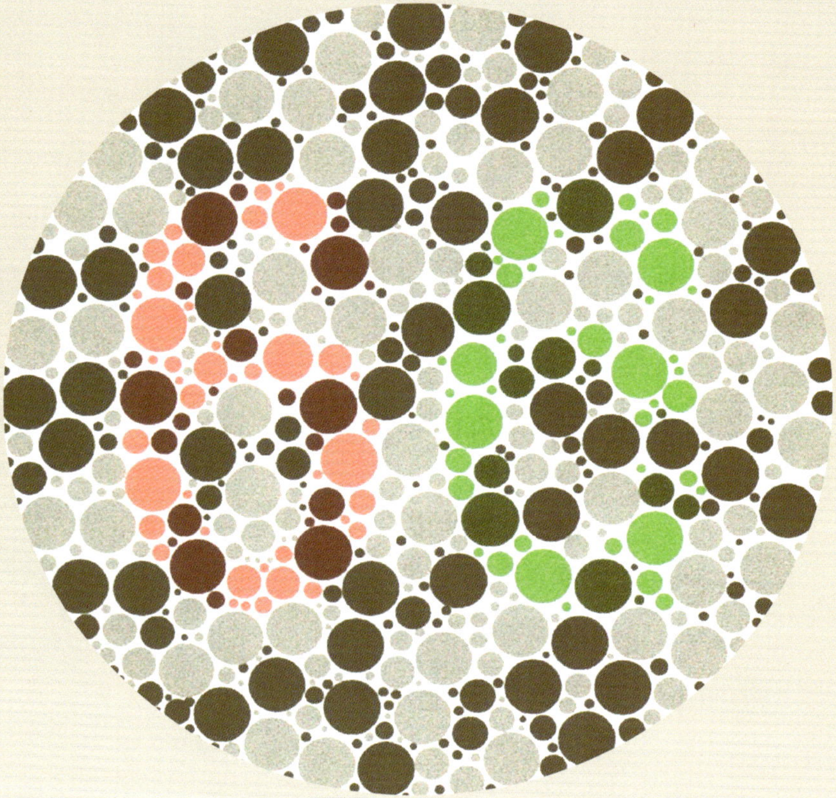

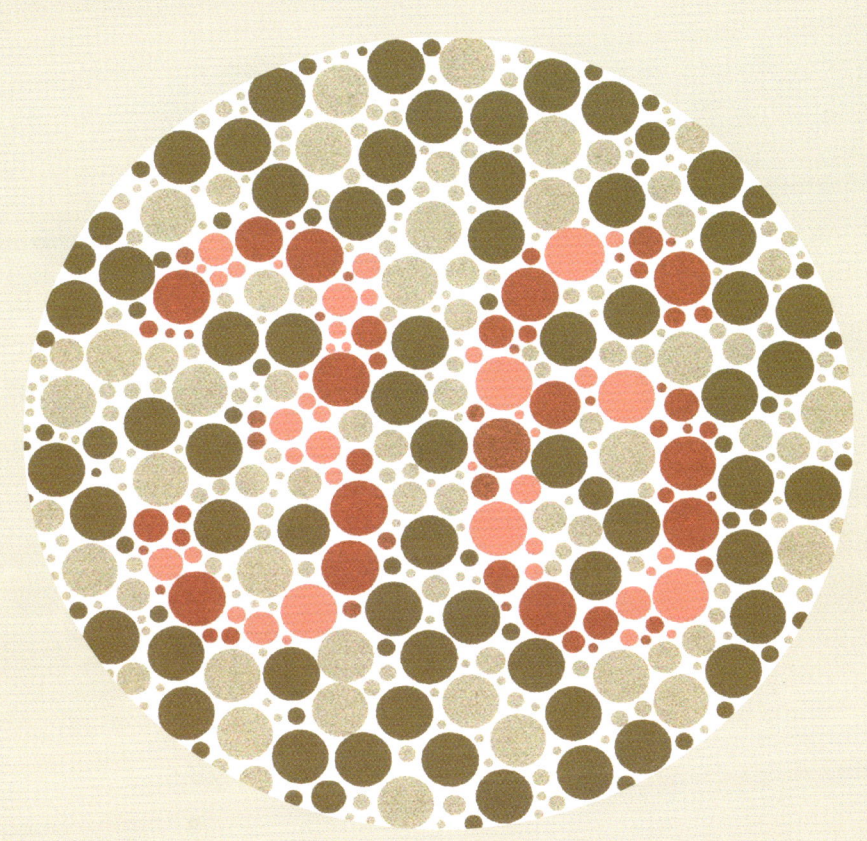

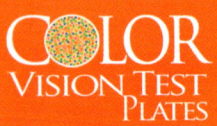

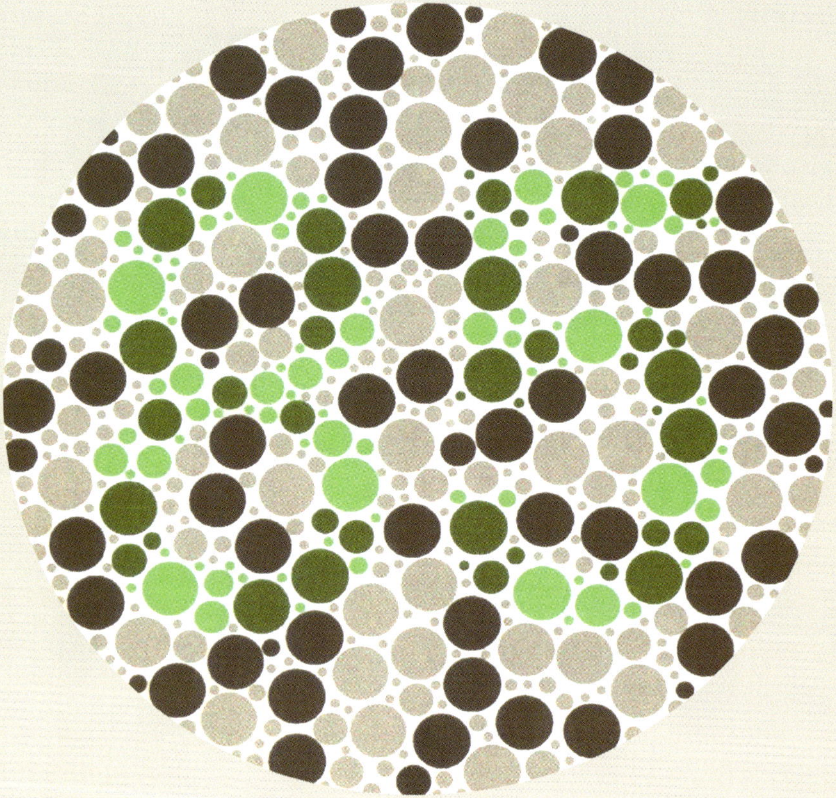

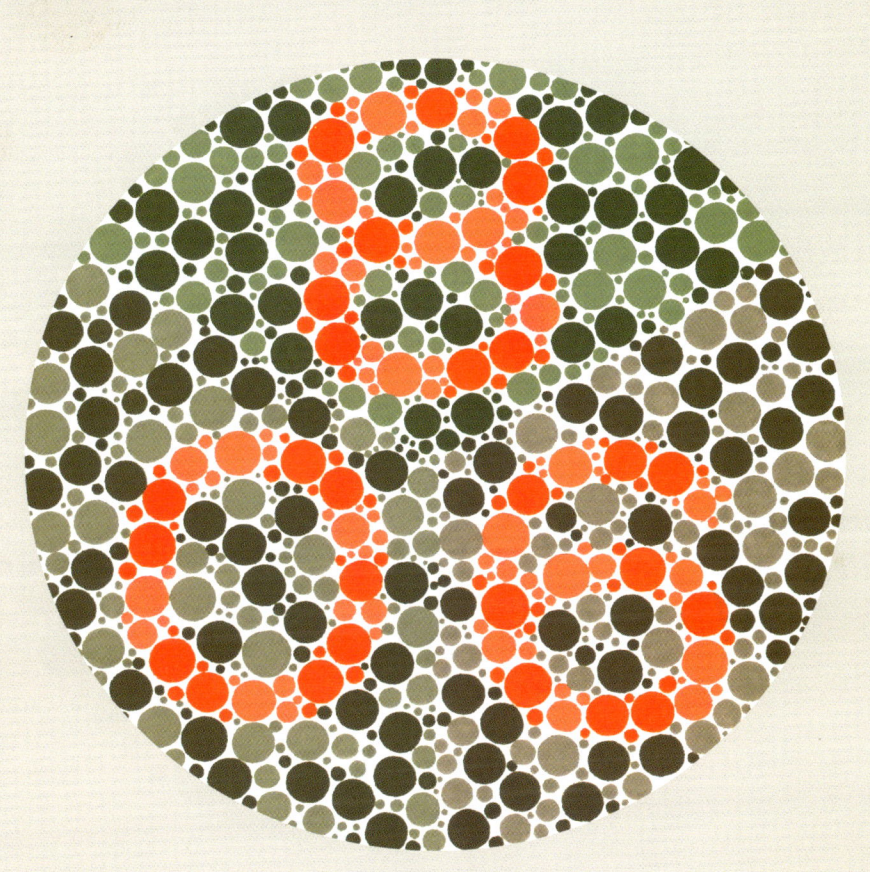

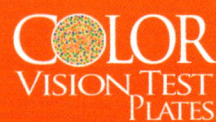

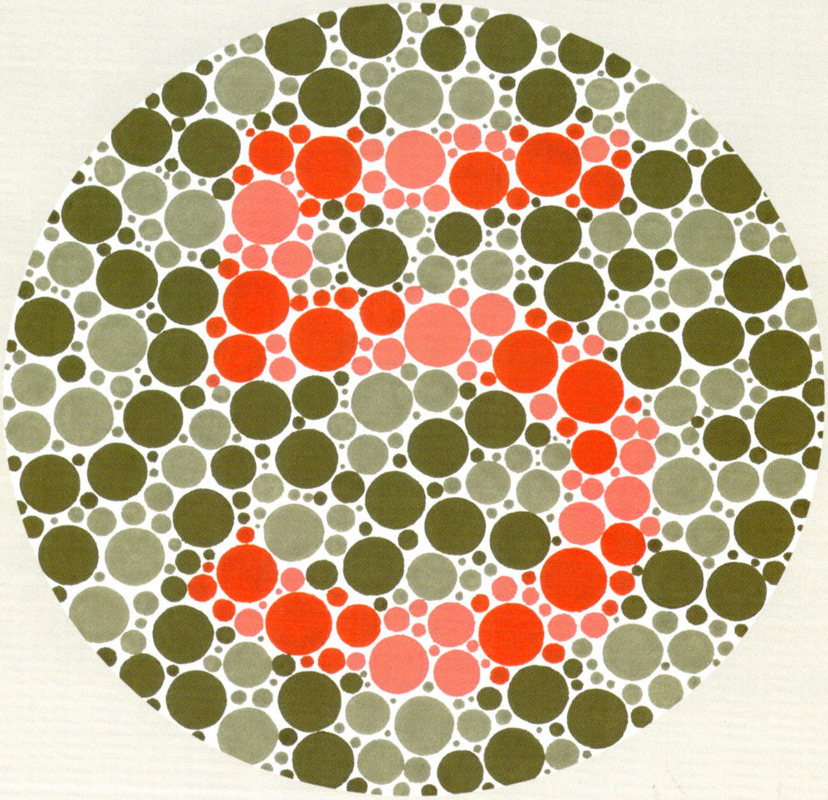

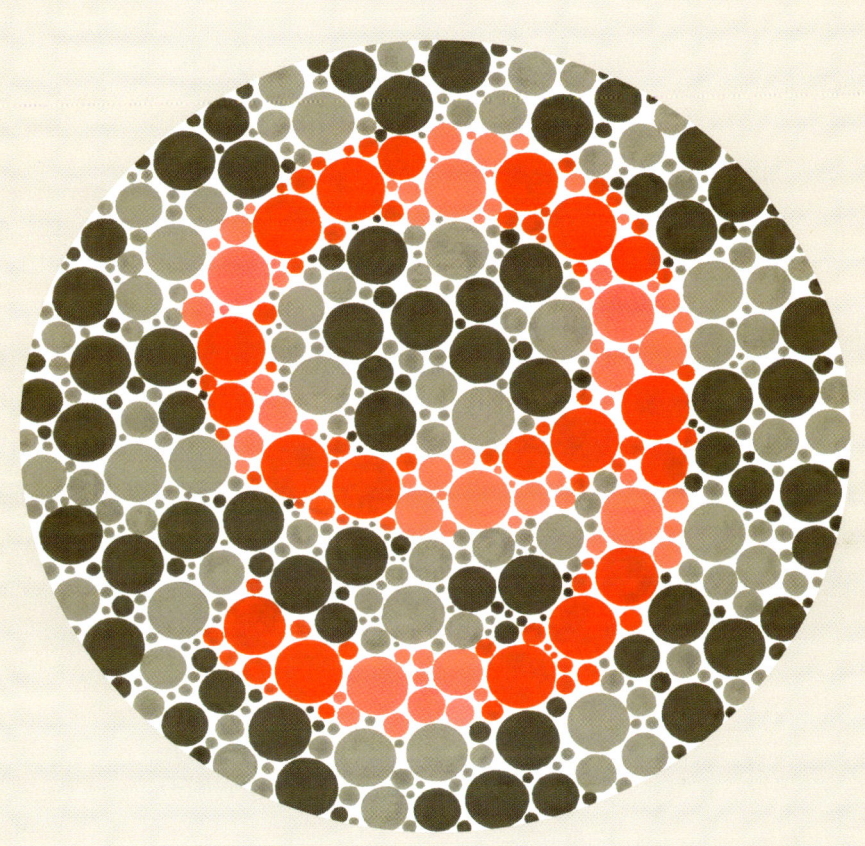

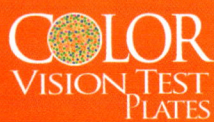

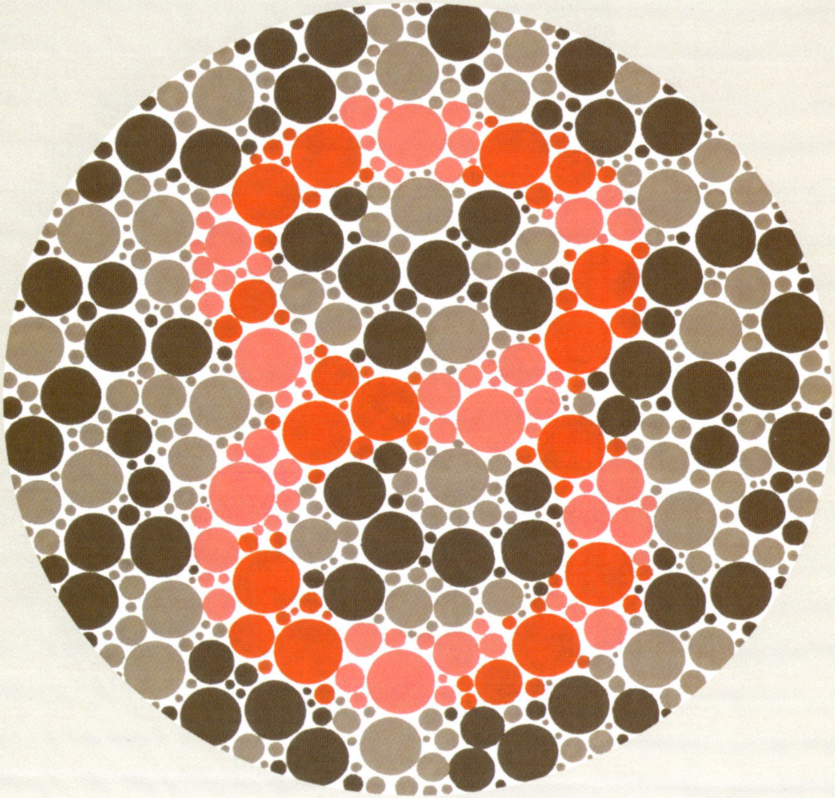

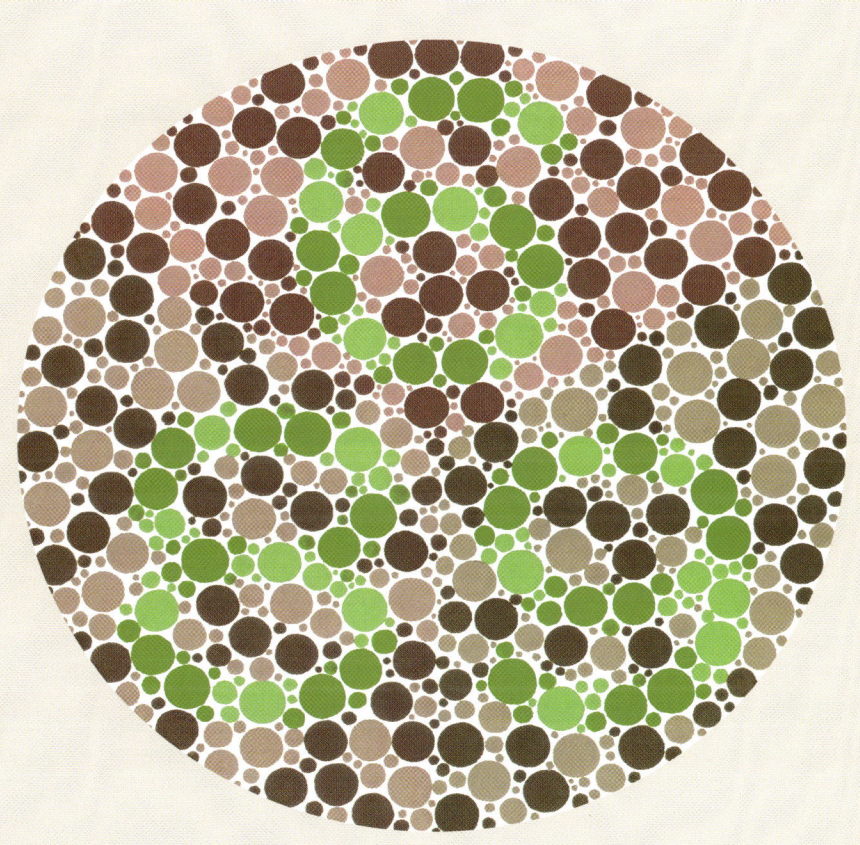

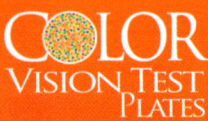

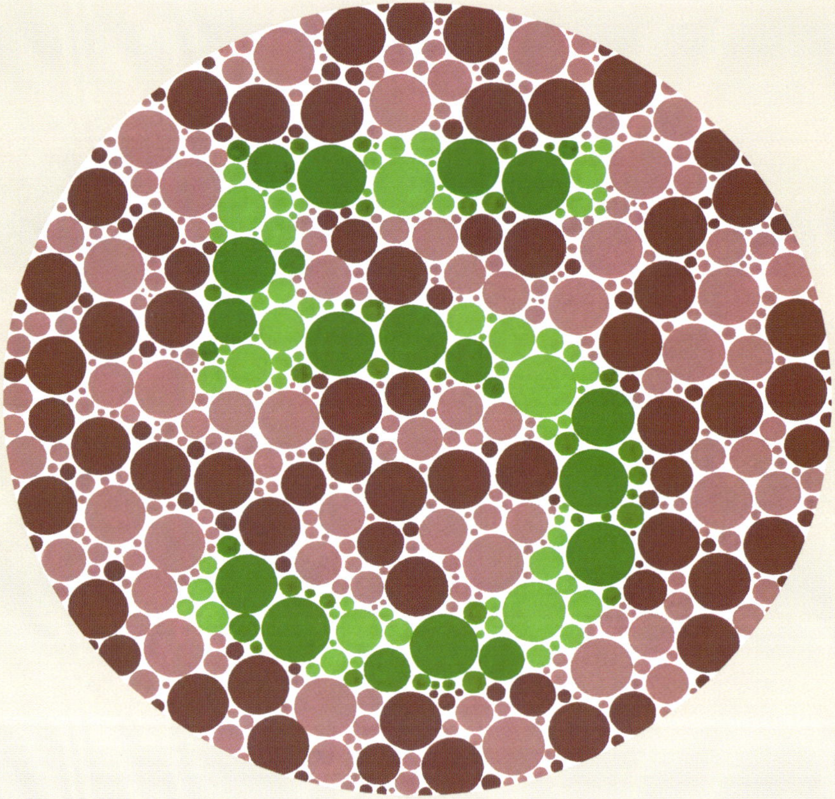

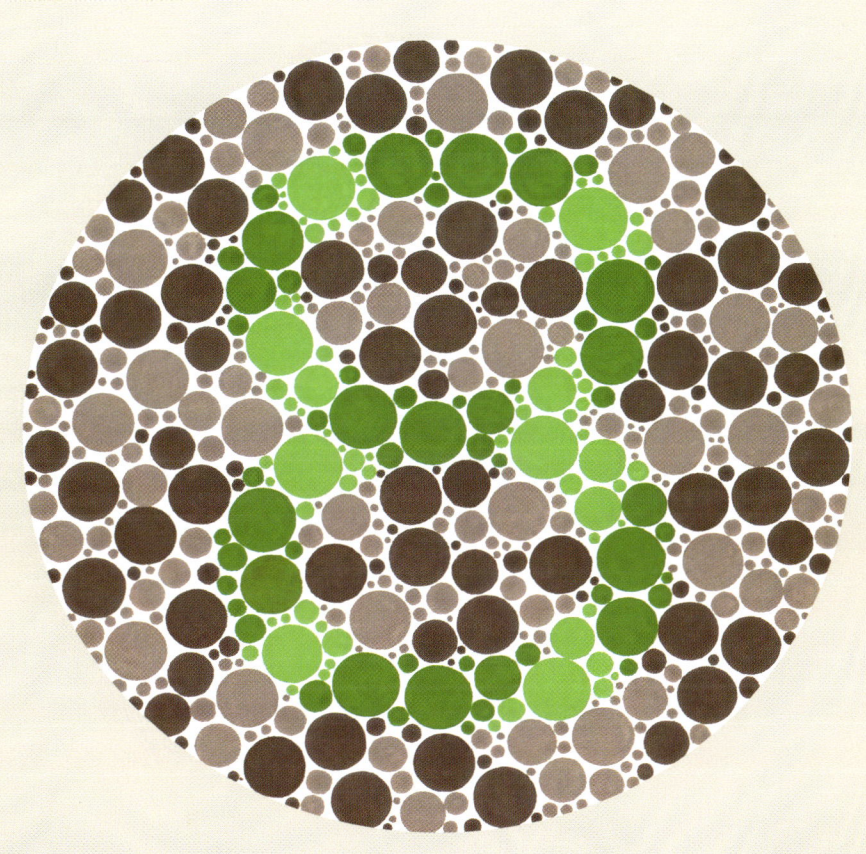

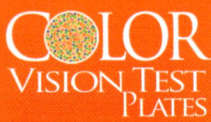

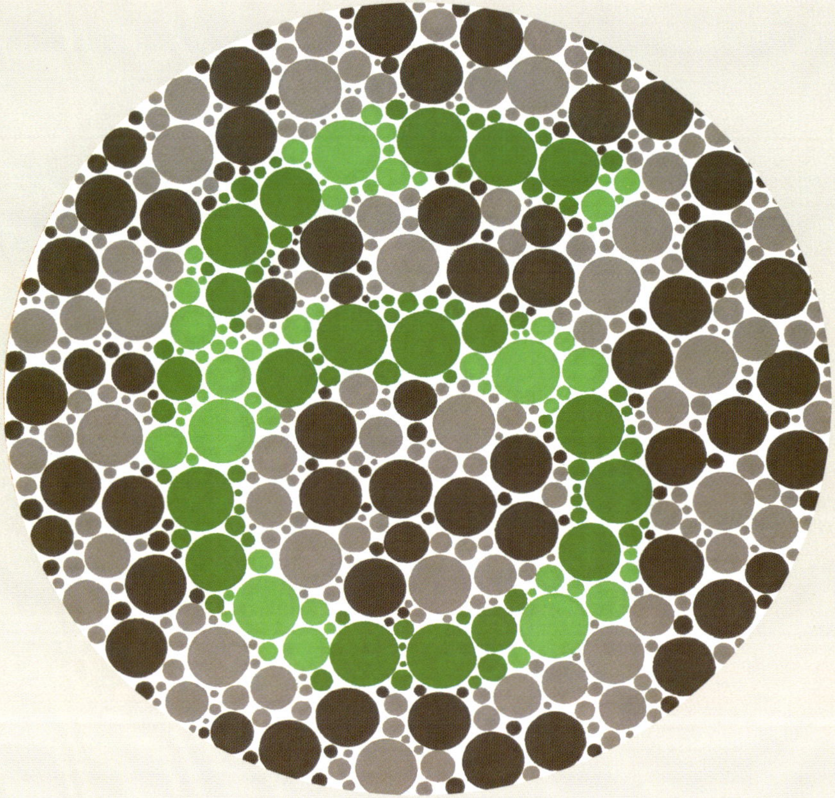

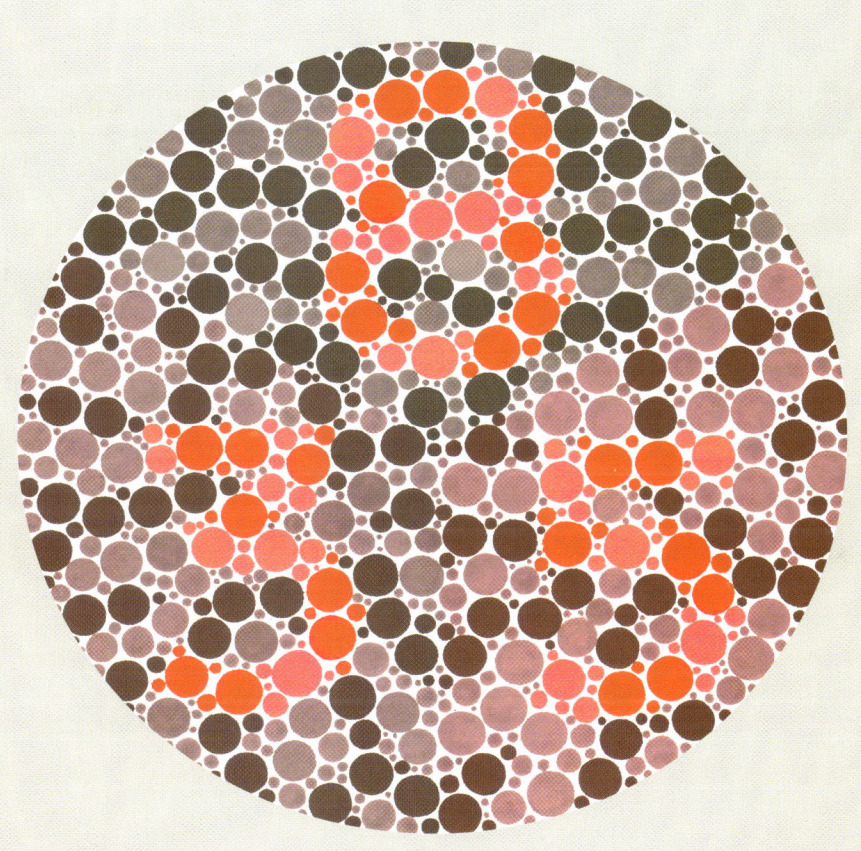

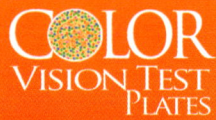

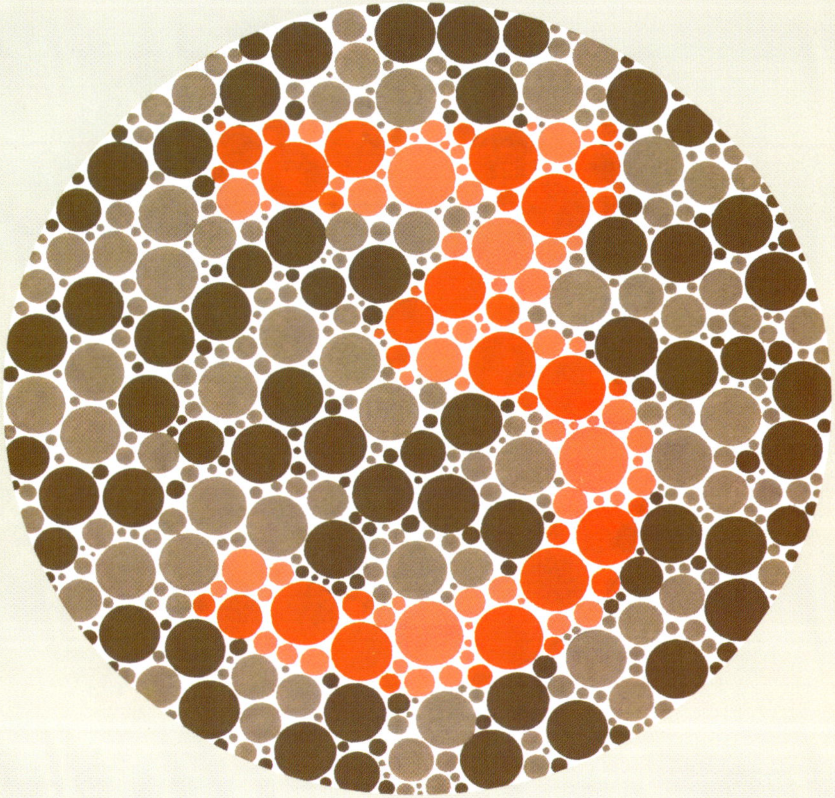

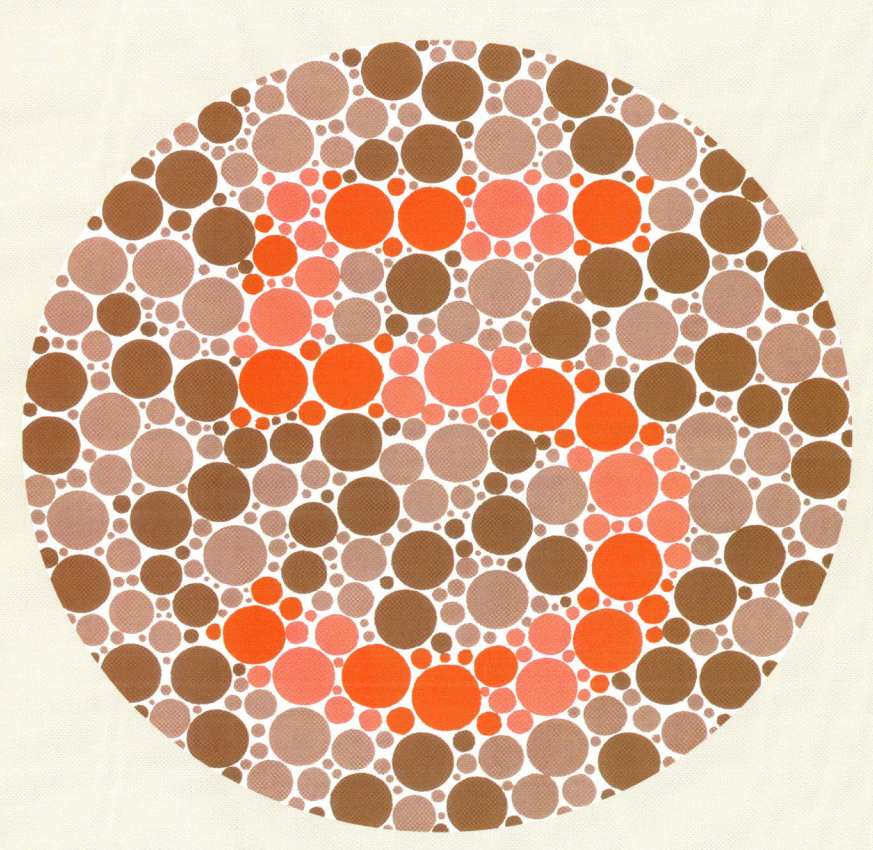

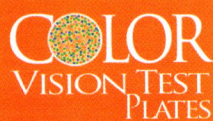

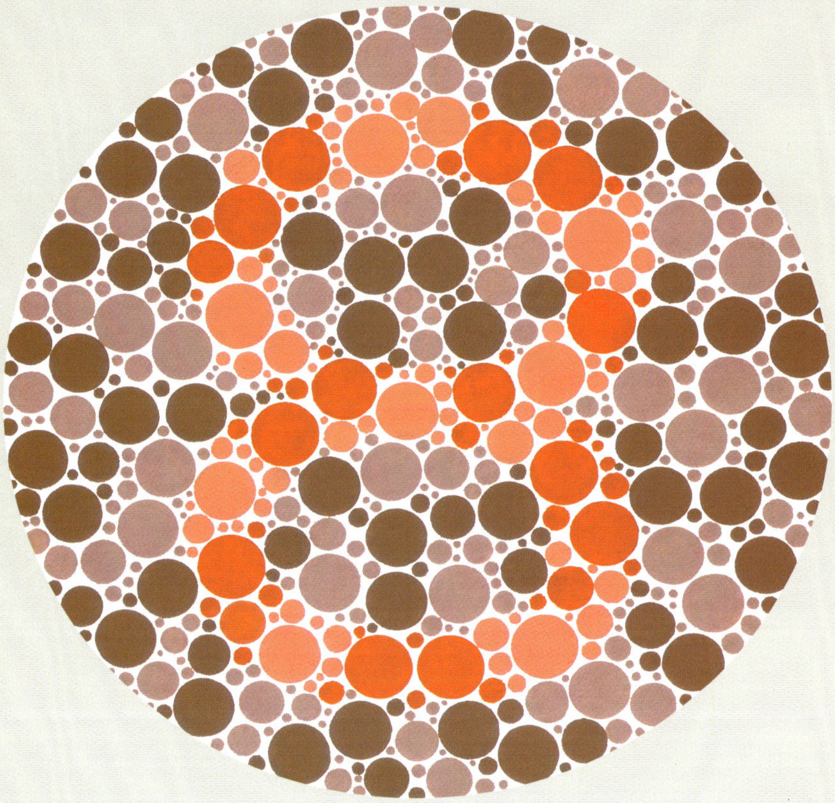

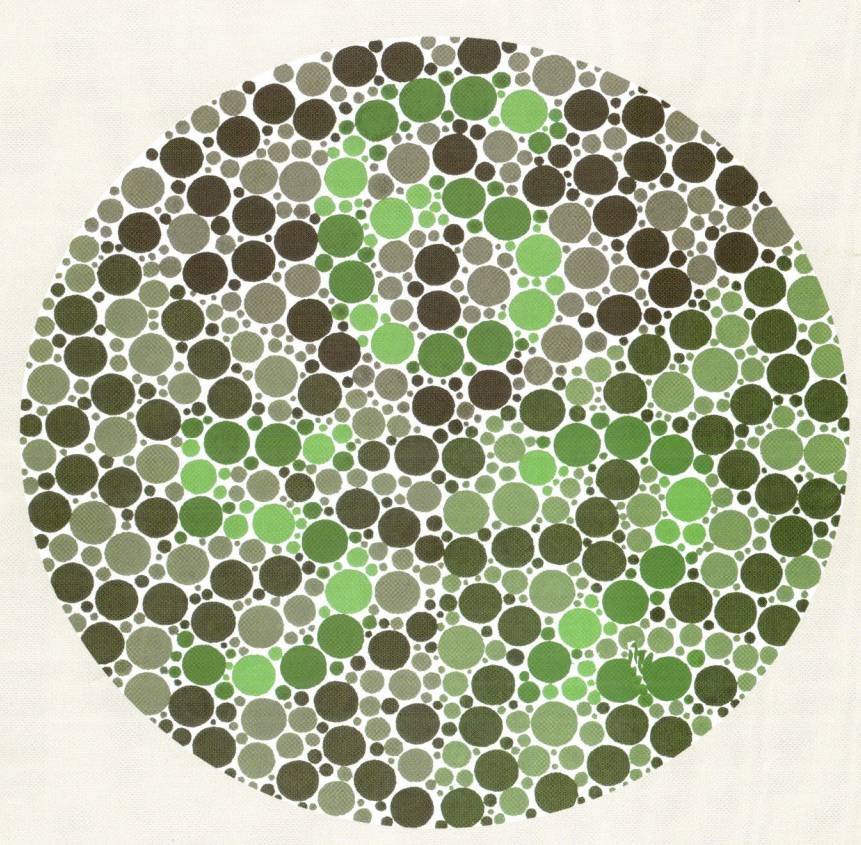

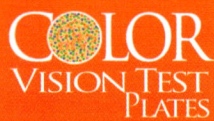

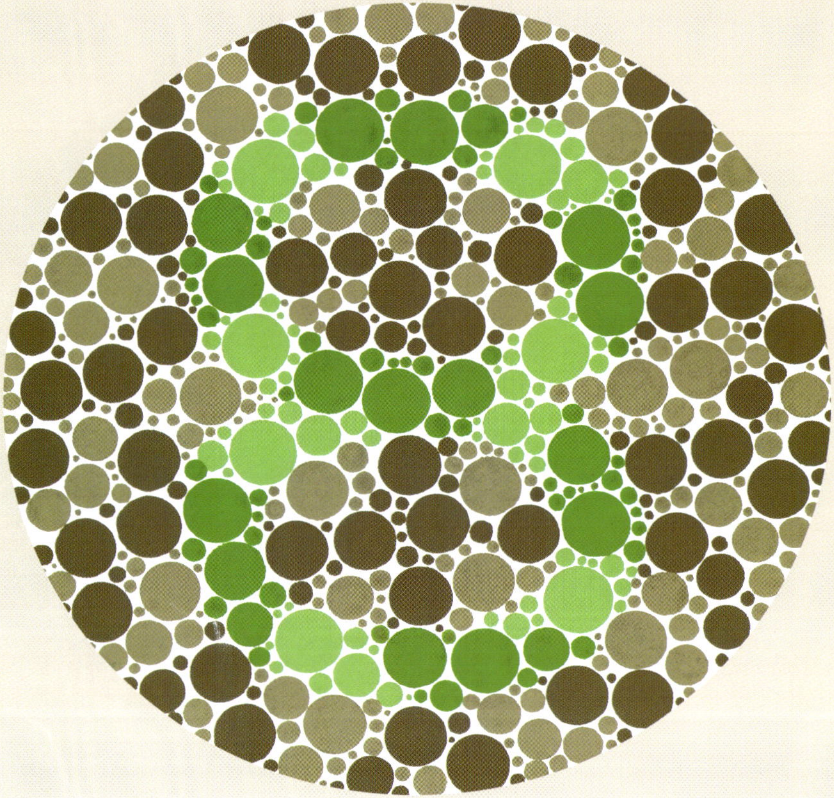

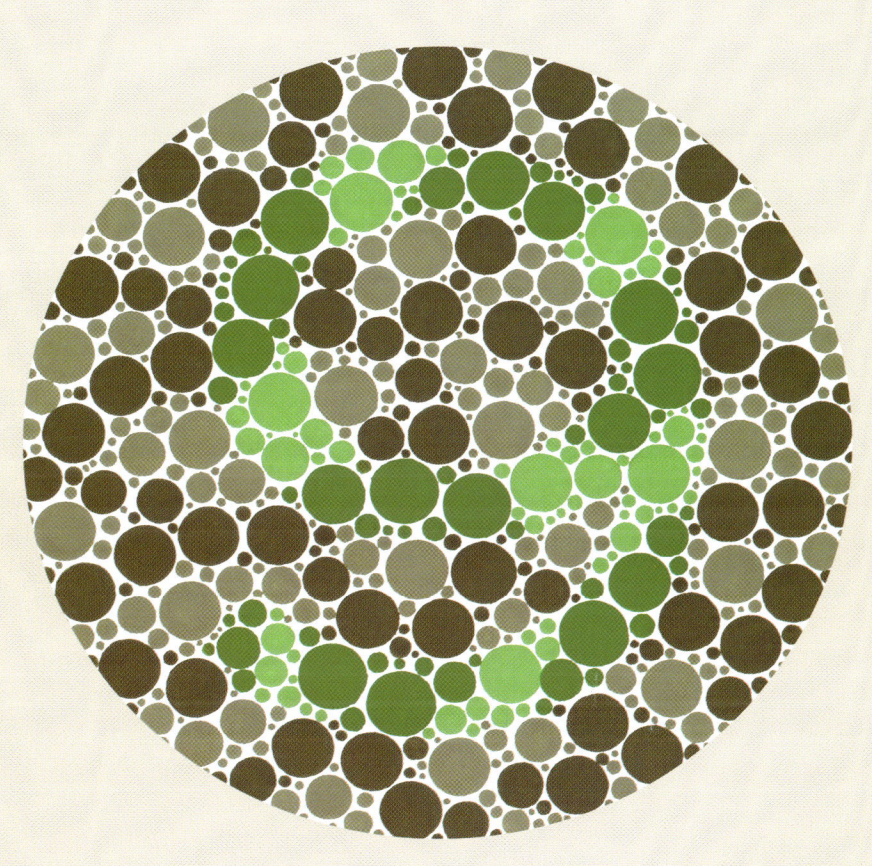

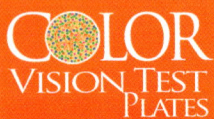

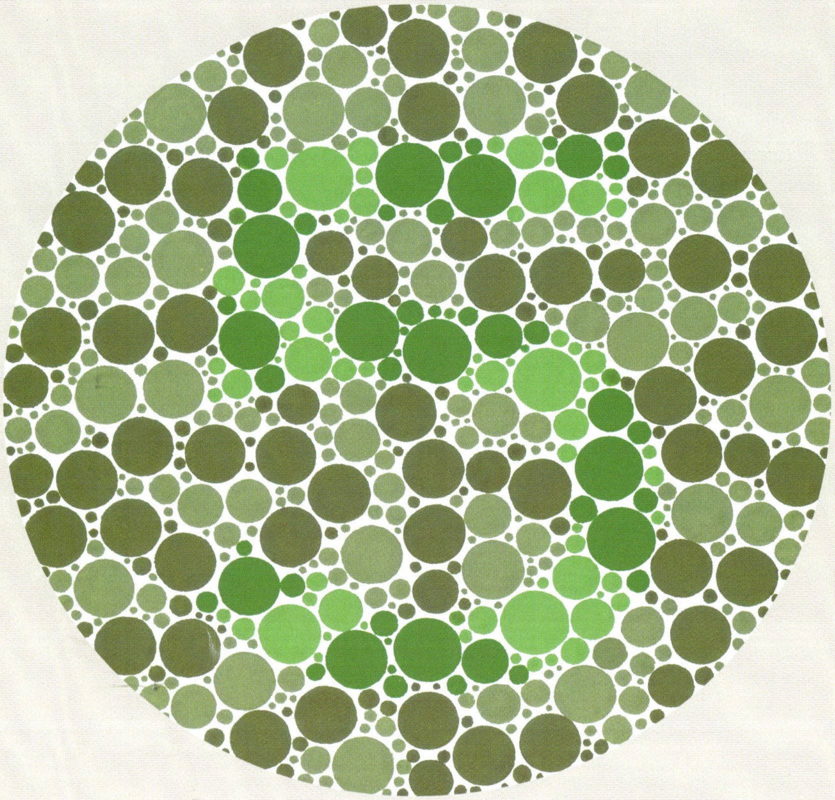

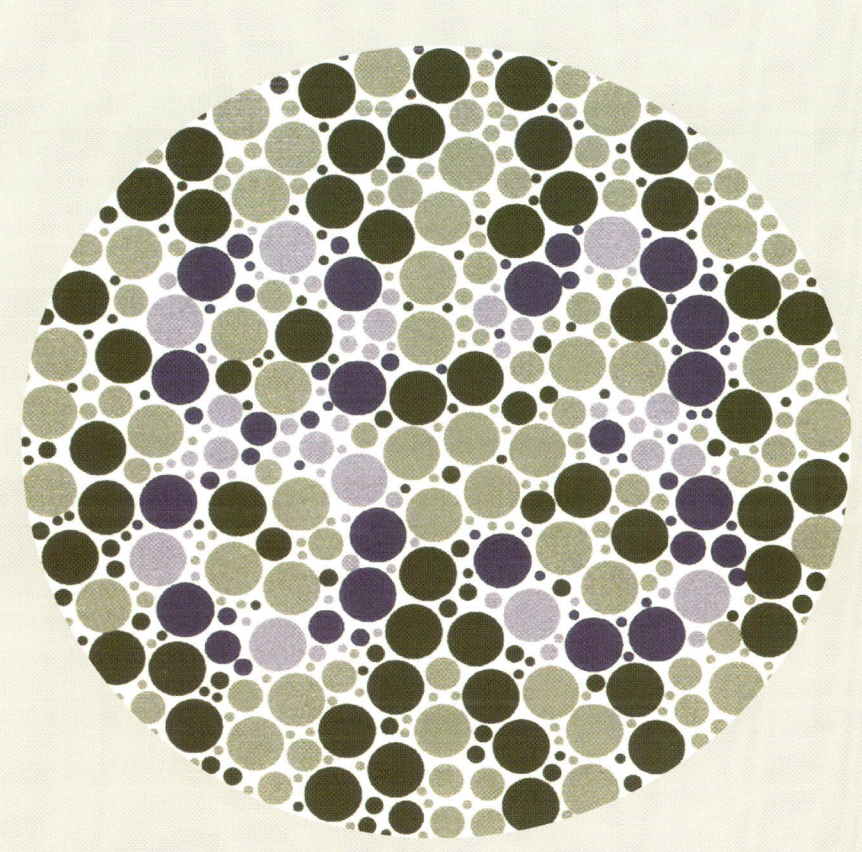

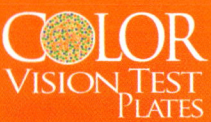

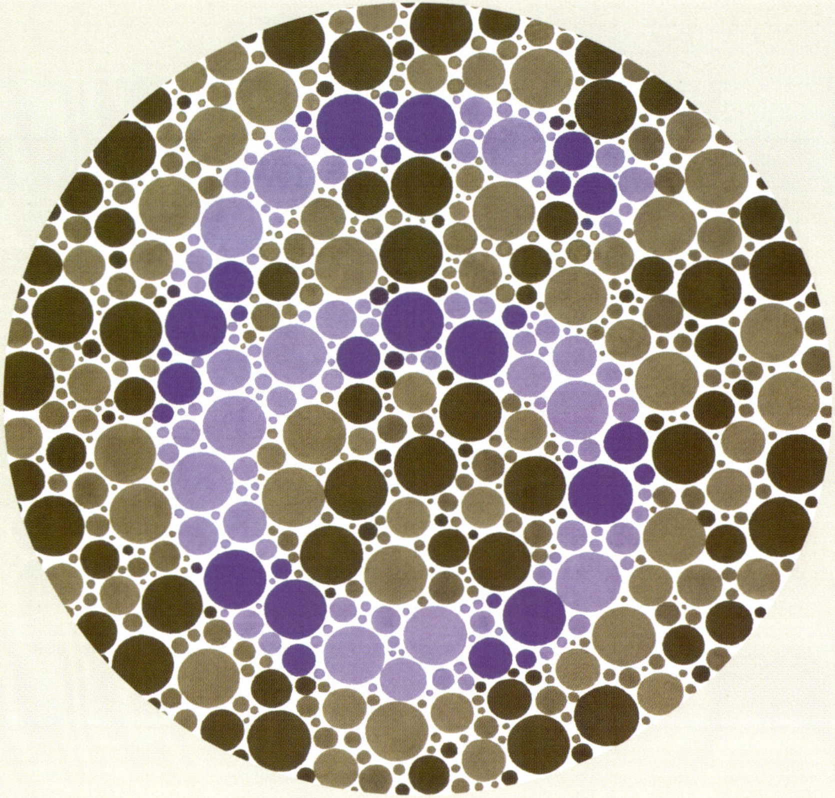

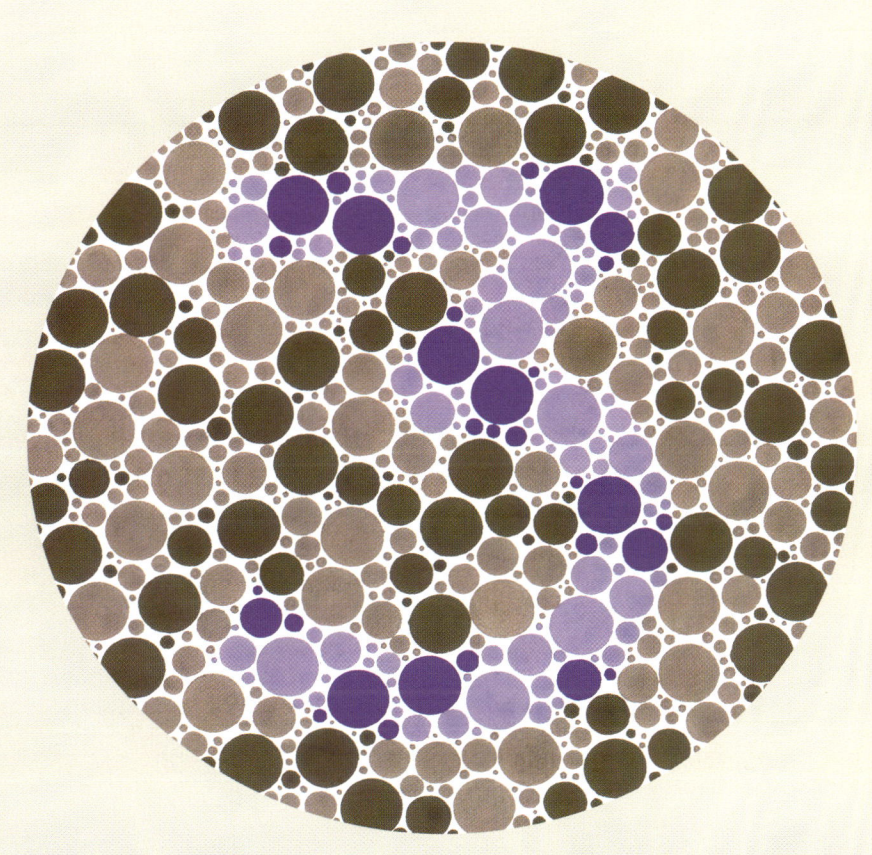

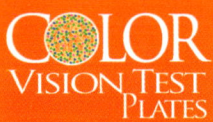

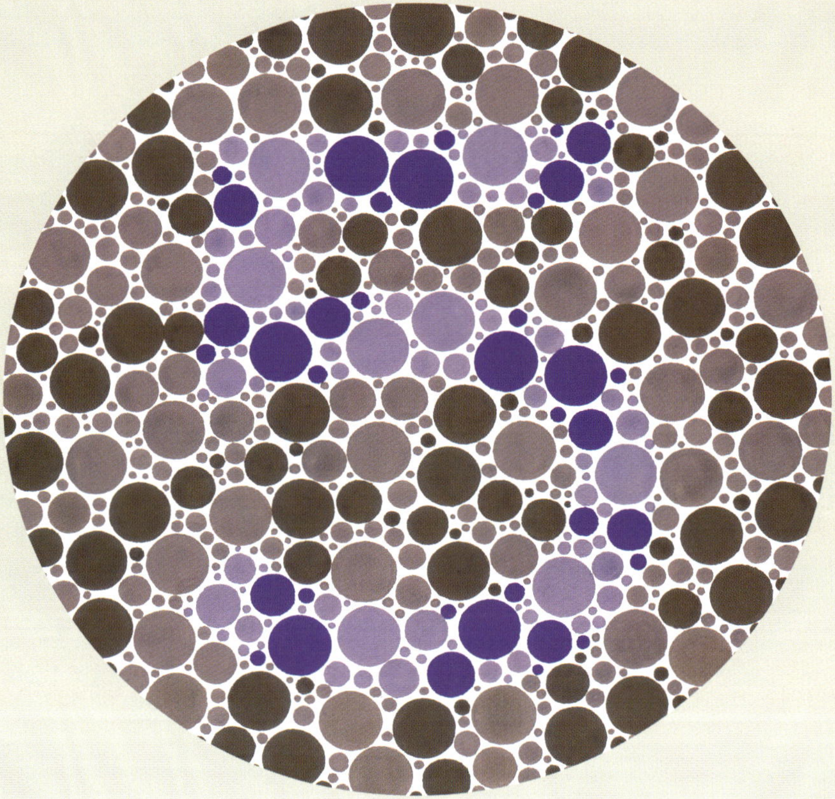

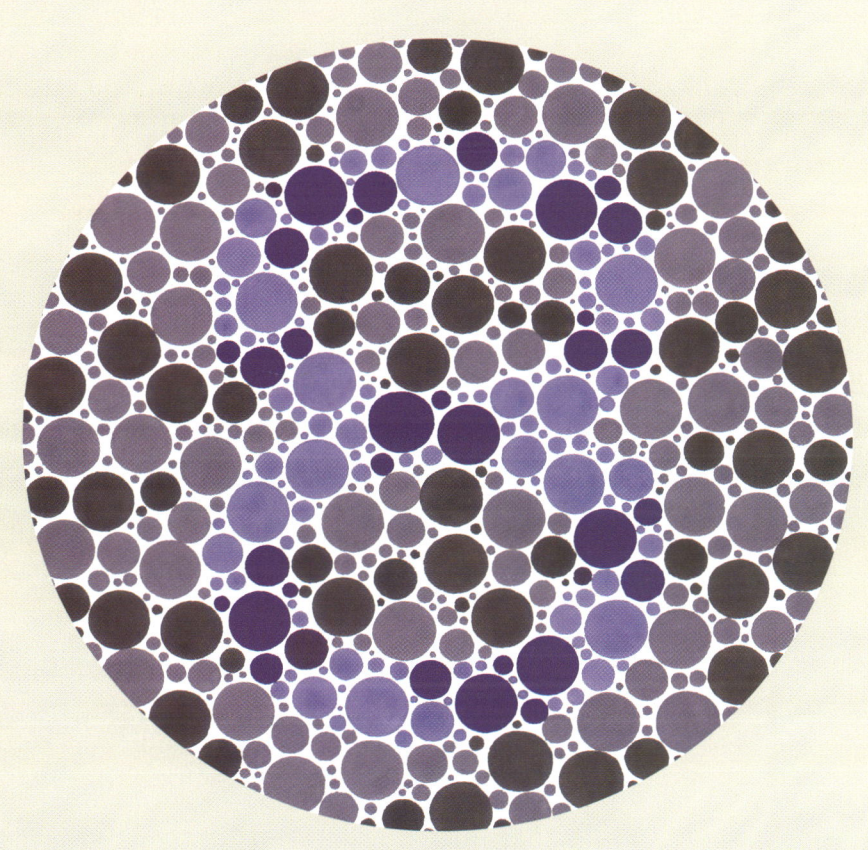

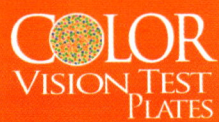

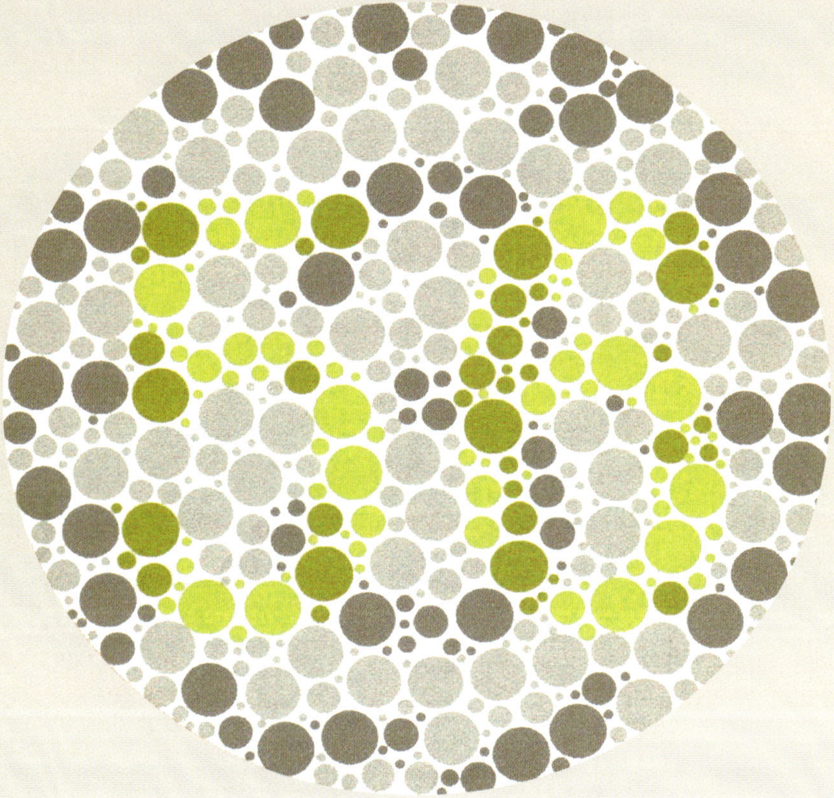

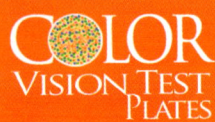

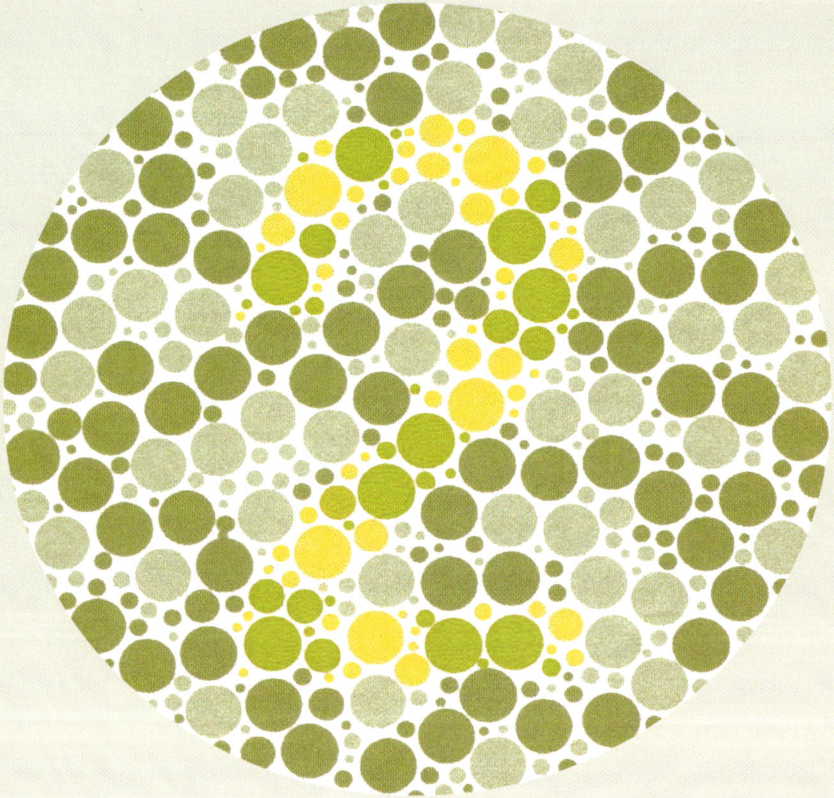

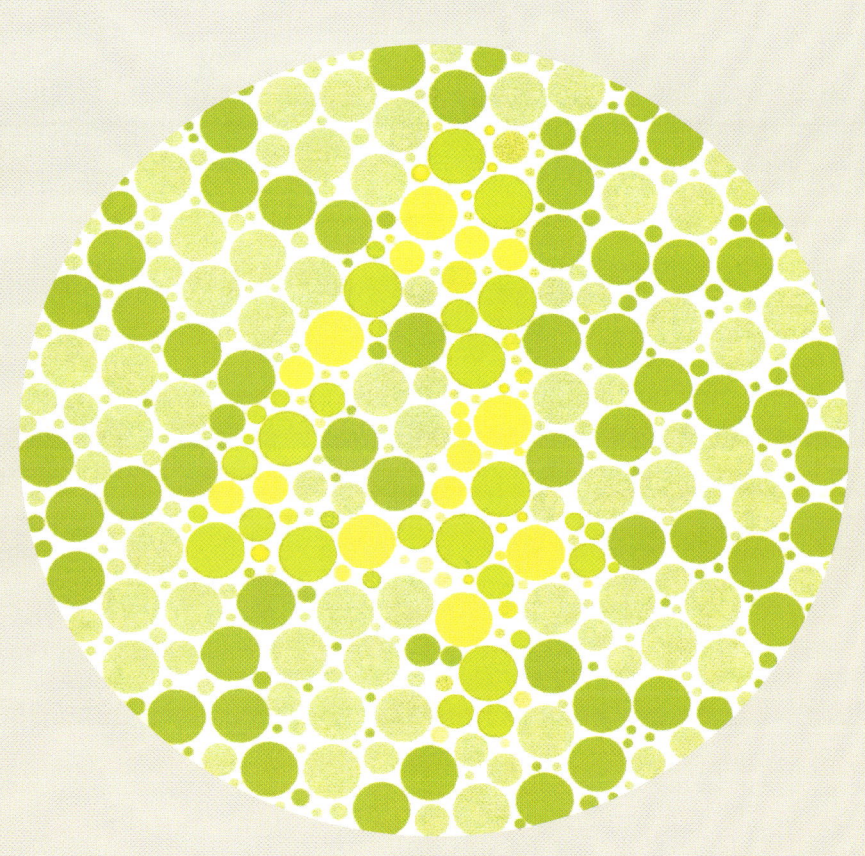

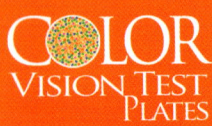

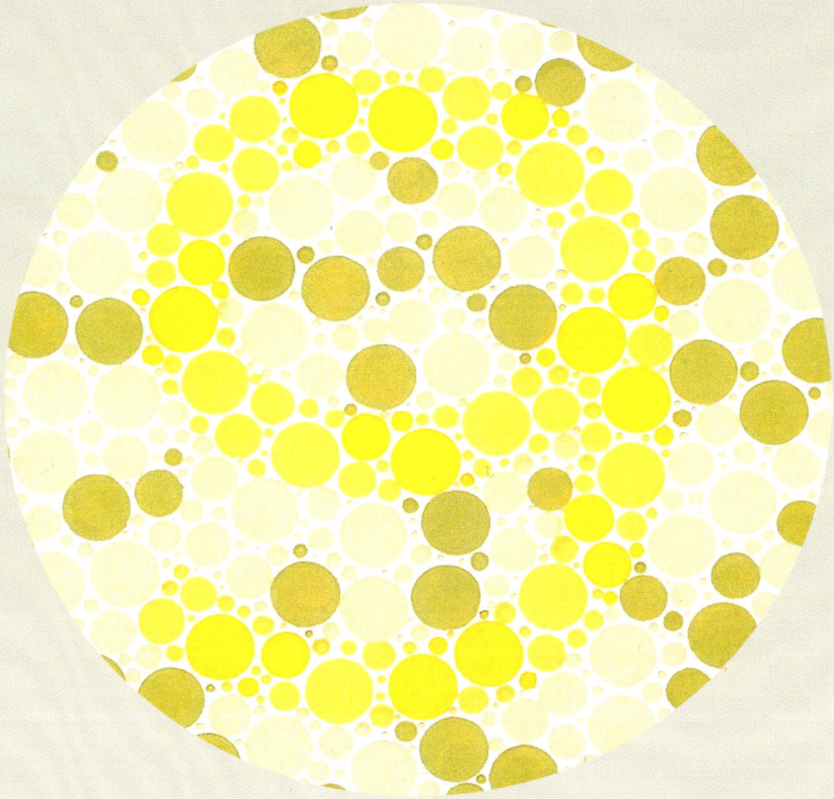

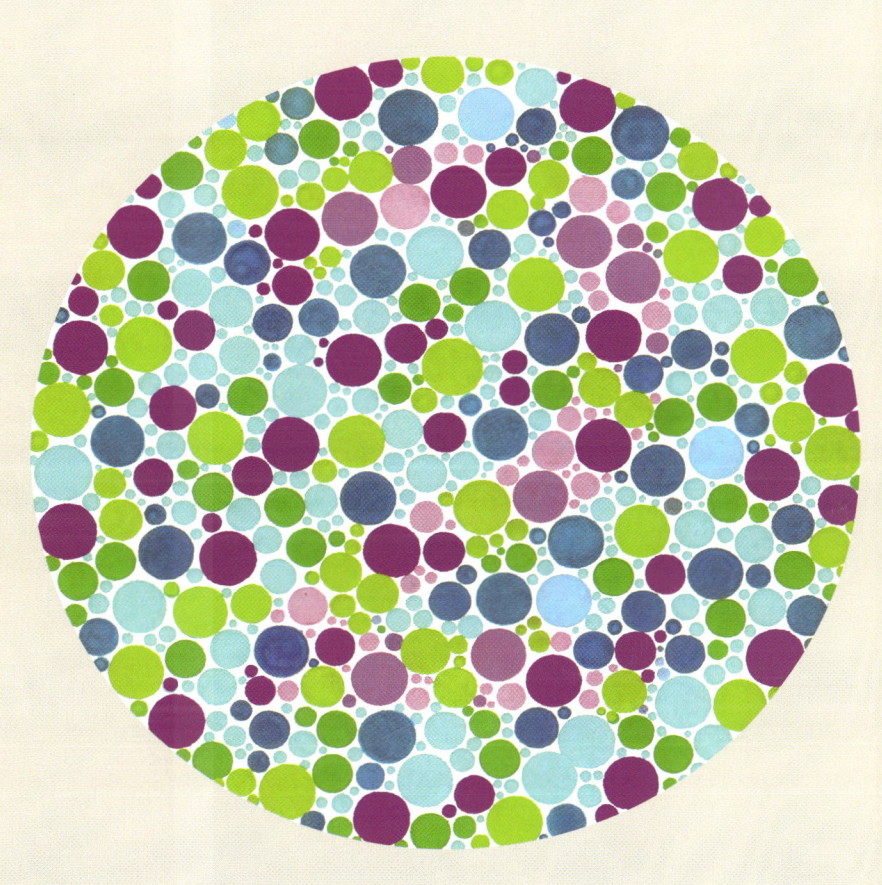

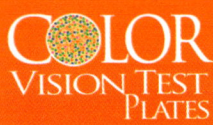

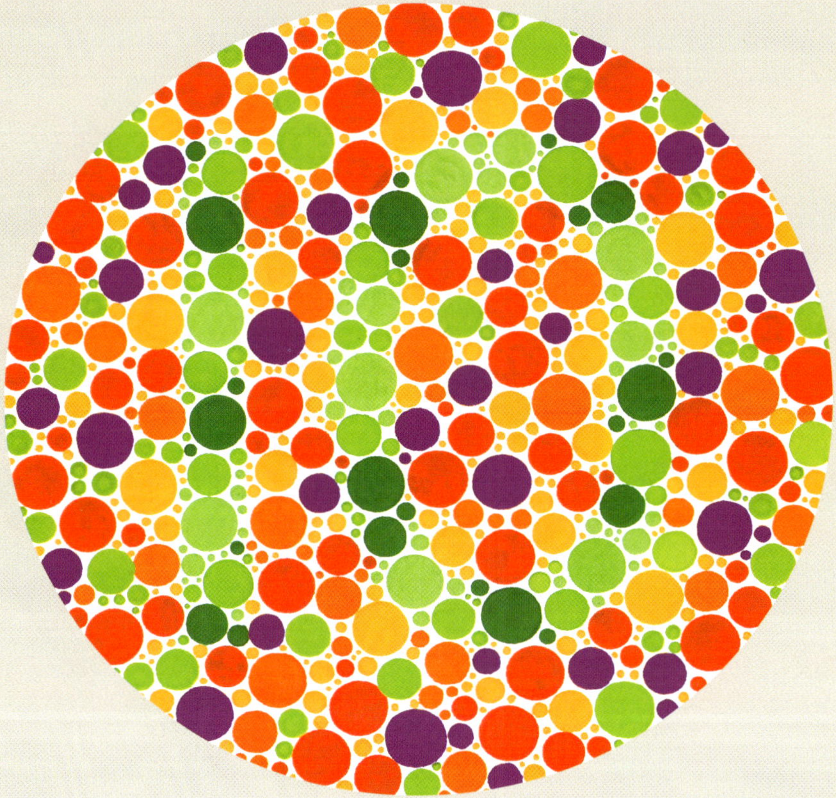

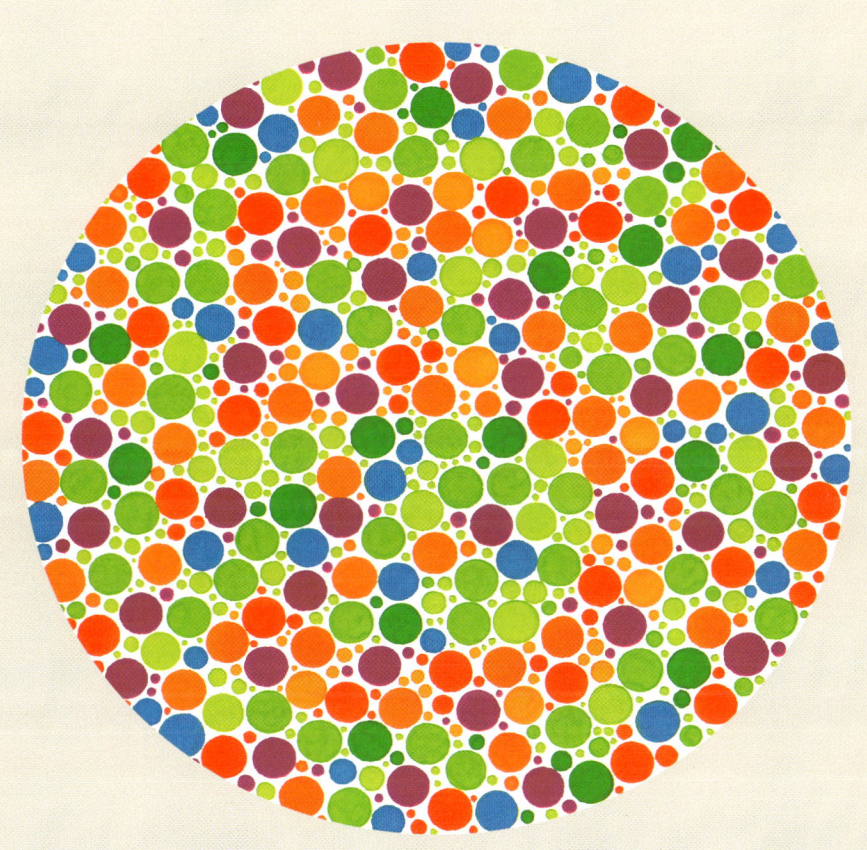

COLOR VISION TEST PLATES

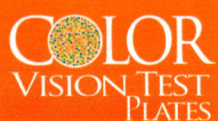

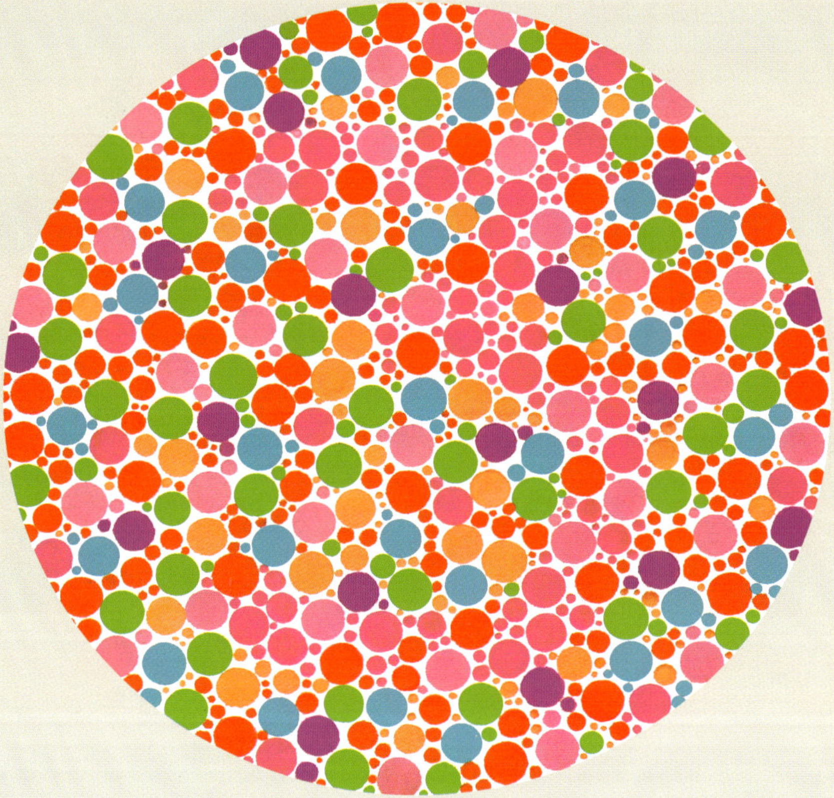

2. Latin letter group

Plate number	Normal	Color vision anomaly		Annotation
		Type	Result	
39	RY	Red-green color vision anomaly	U	Distinguish red, green color blindness, and a part of red-green weakness
		Red color vision anomaly	Y	
		Green color vision anomaly	R	
40	P	Red color vision anomaly	N	Distinguish red color blindness, and a part of red weakness
41	E	Green color vision anomaly	T	Distinguish green color blindness, and a part of green weakness
42	M	Green color vision anomaly	Can't read it	
43	B	Red blindness	Can't read it	Distinguish red blindness
44	W	Green blindness	Can't read it	Distinguish green blindness
45	A	Red color vision anomaly	Can't read it	
46	BE	Red-green color vision anomaly	S	Distinguish red, green color blindness, and a part of red-green weakness
		Red color vision anomaly	E	
		Green color vision anomaly	B	

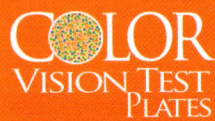

continued

Plate number	Normal	Color vision anomaly		Annotation
		Type	Result	
47	F	Blue (violet) color vision anomaly	Can't read it	Distinguish blue (violet) blindness
48	K	Blue (violet) color vision anomaly	Can't read it	Distinguish blue (violet) weakness
49	V	Yellow blindness	Can't read it	Distinguish yellow blindness
50	D	Strong degree of yellow weakness	Can't read it	Distinguish yellow weakness
51	H	Mild degree of yellow weakness	Can't read it	Distinguish yellow weakness

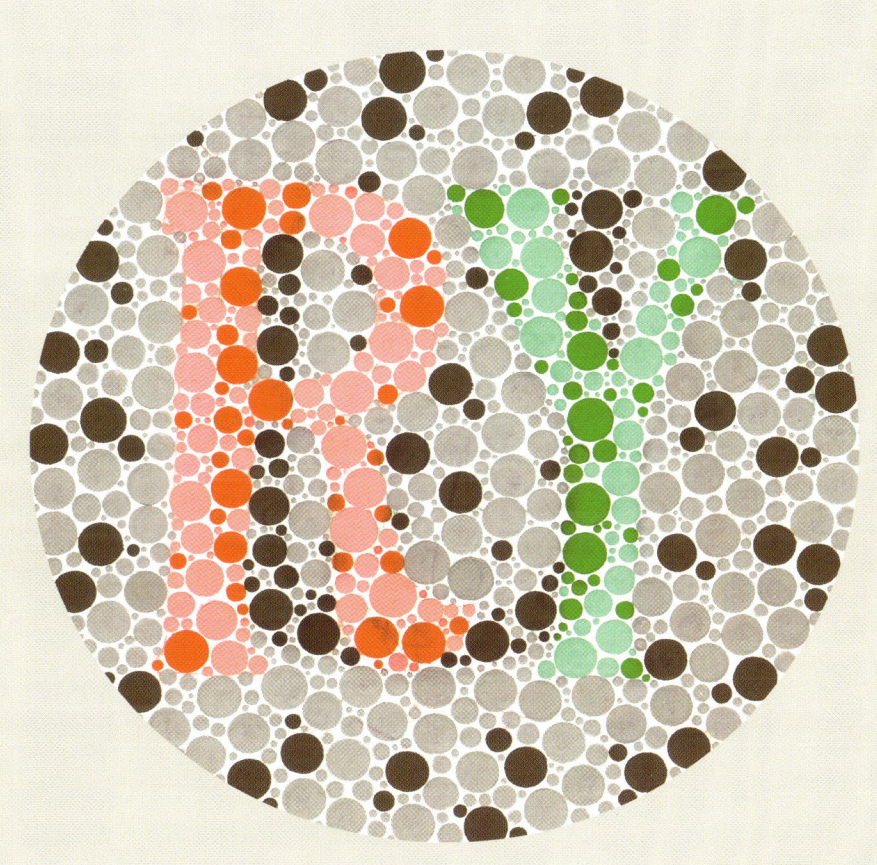

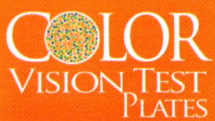
COLOR
VISION TEST
PLATES

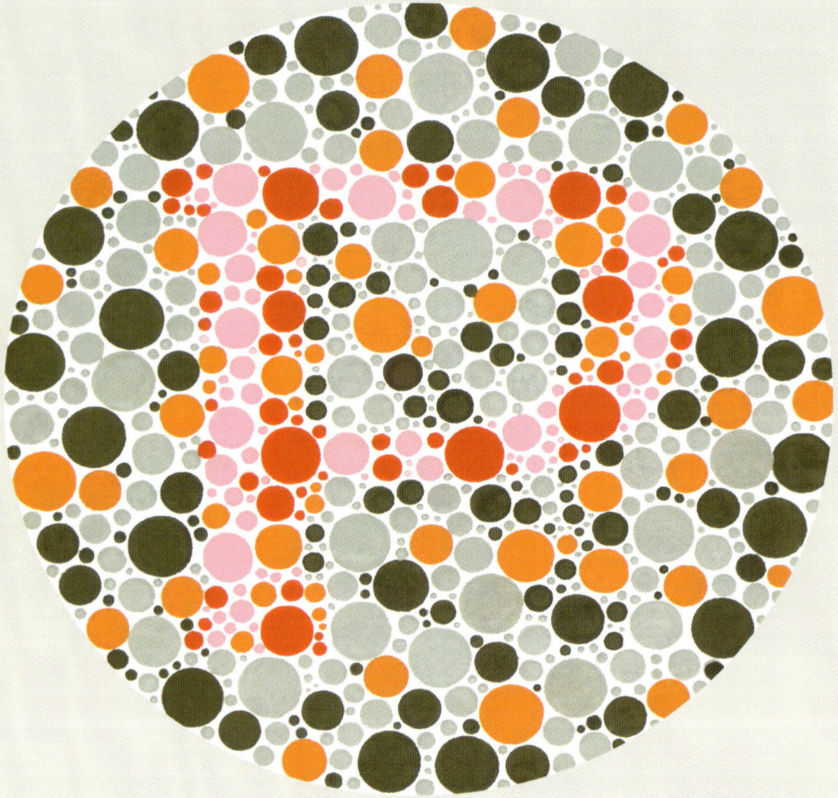

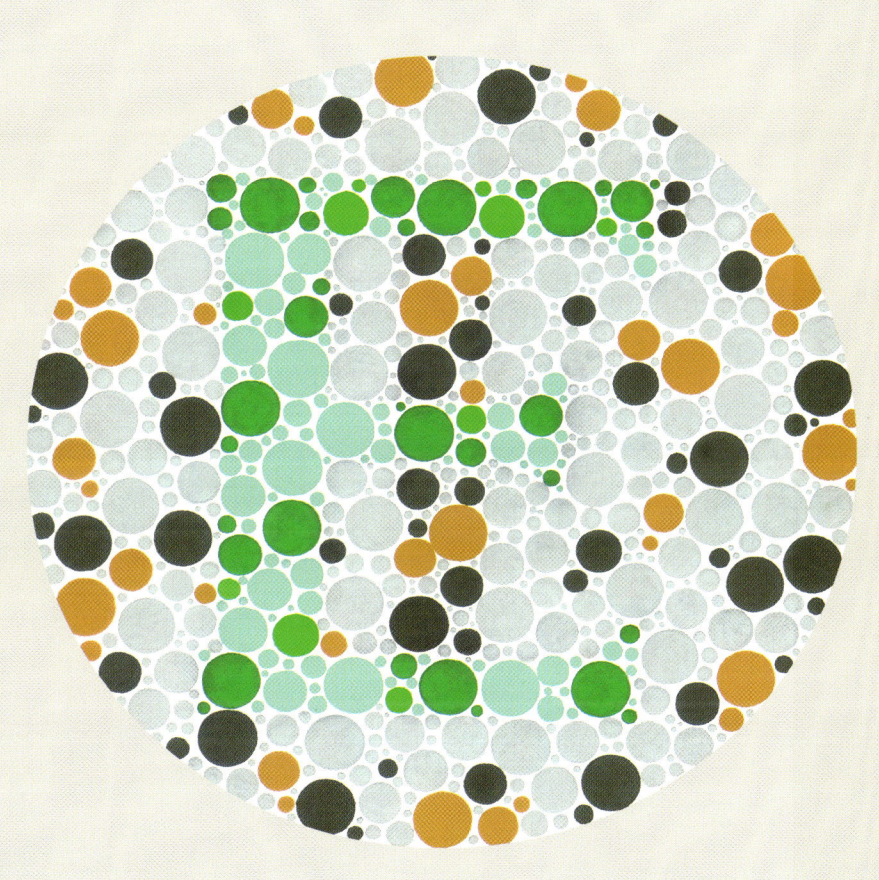

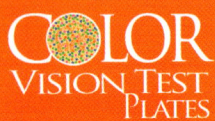

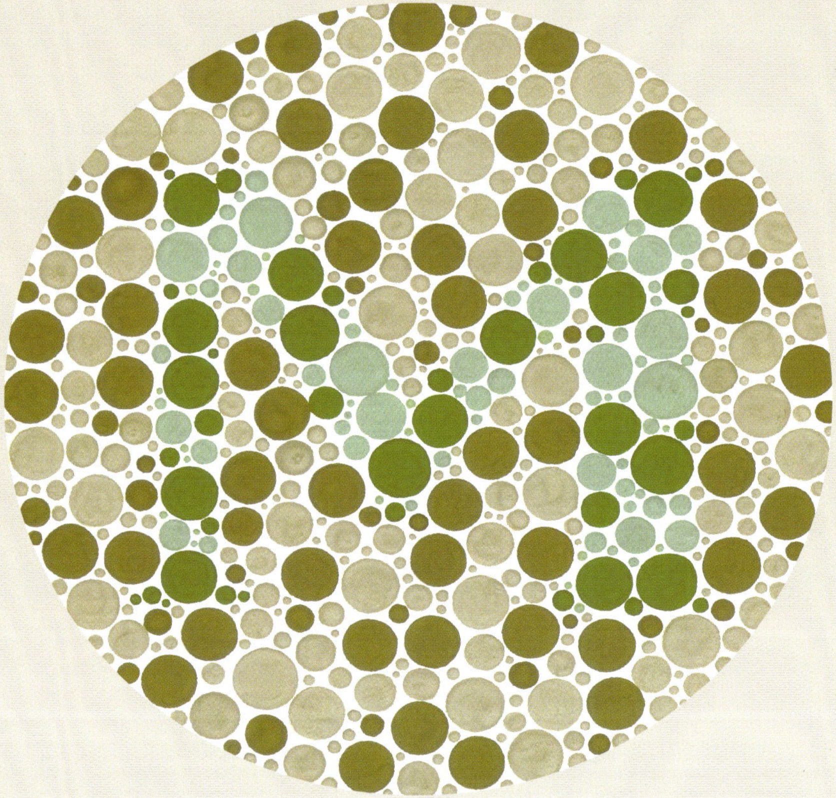

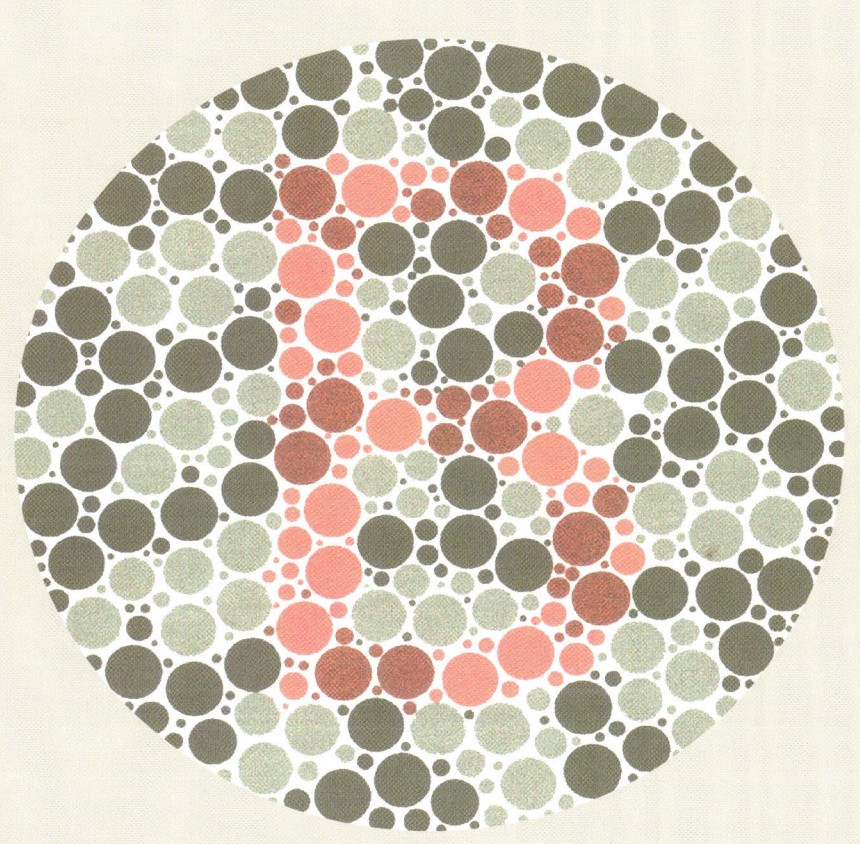

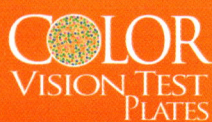

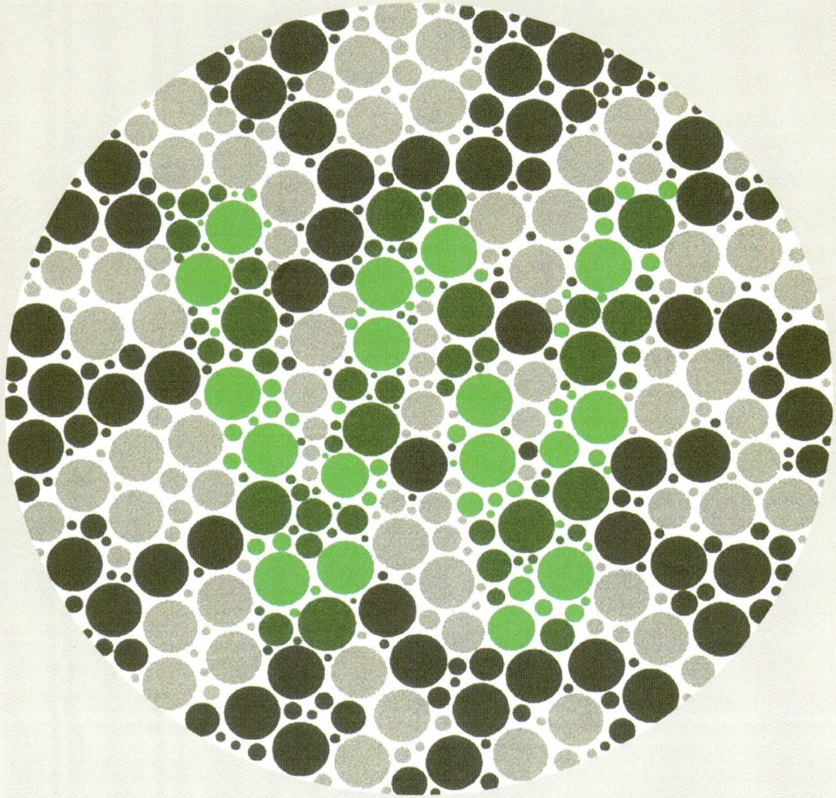

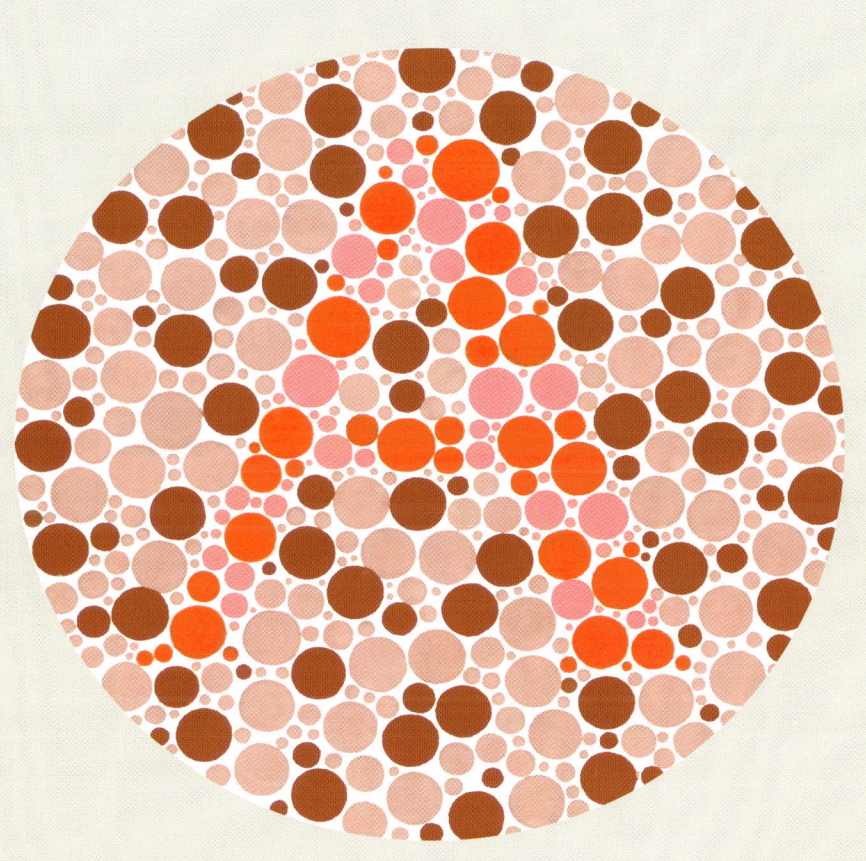

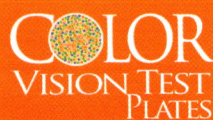

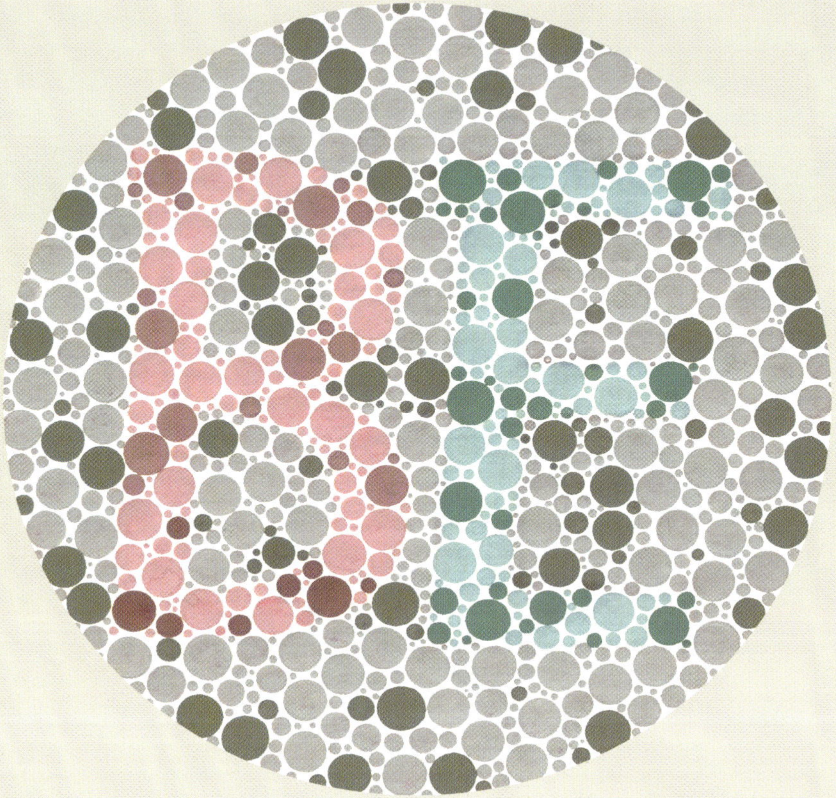

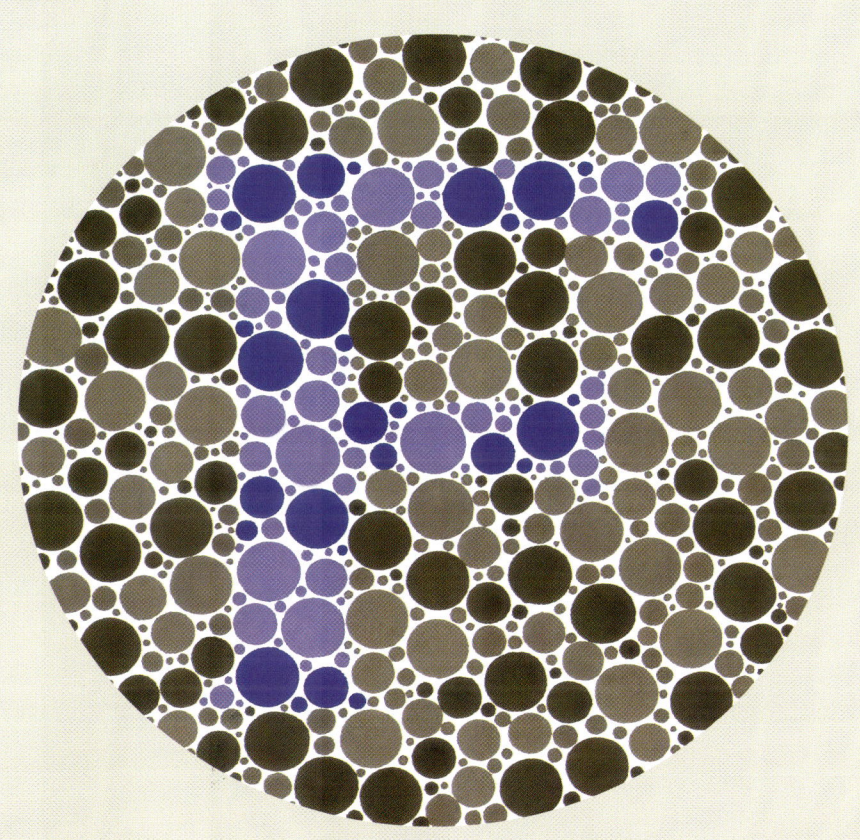

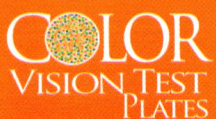

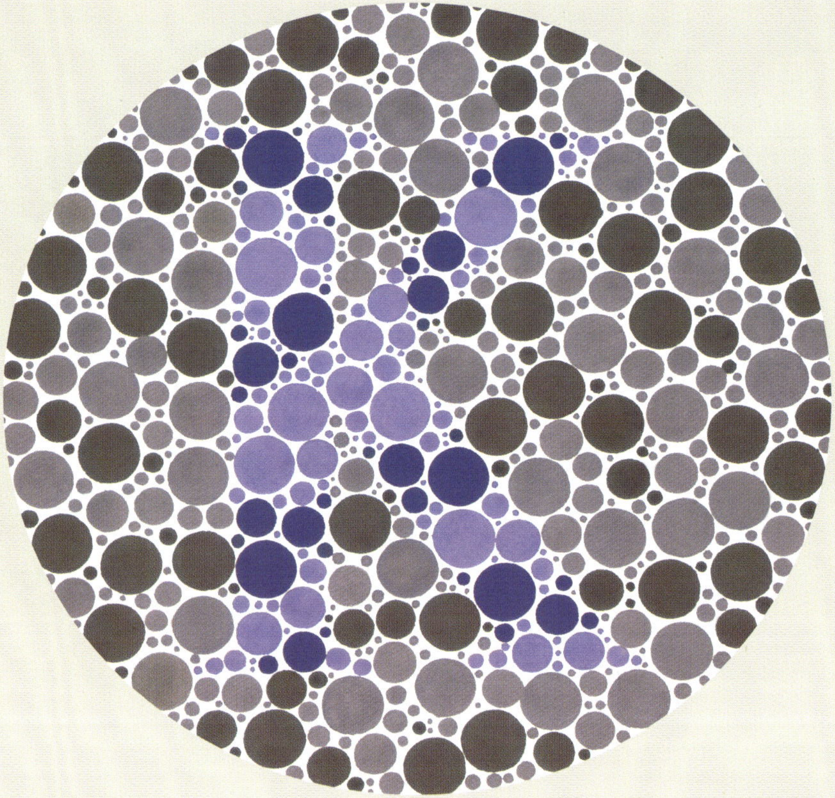

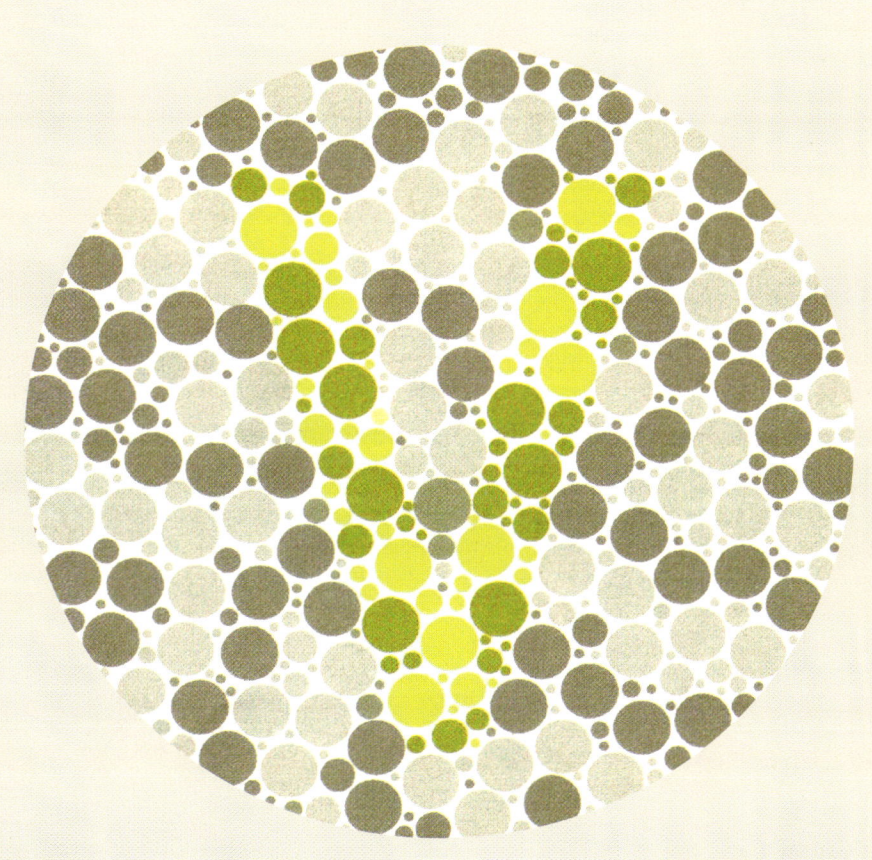

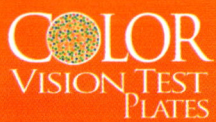

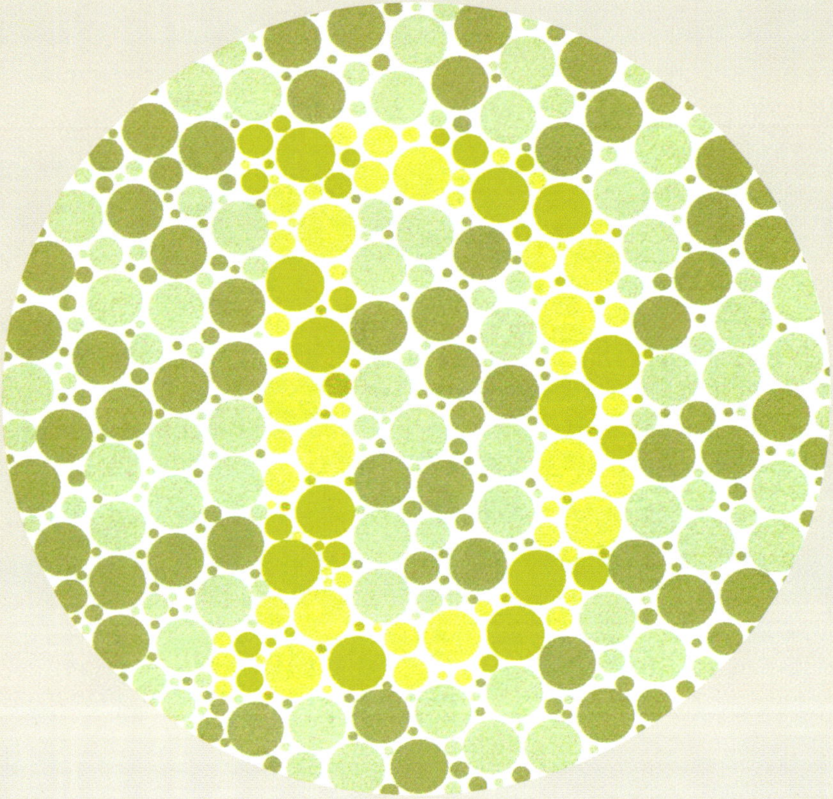

COLOR
VISION TEST
PLATES

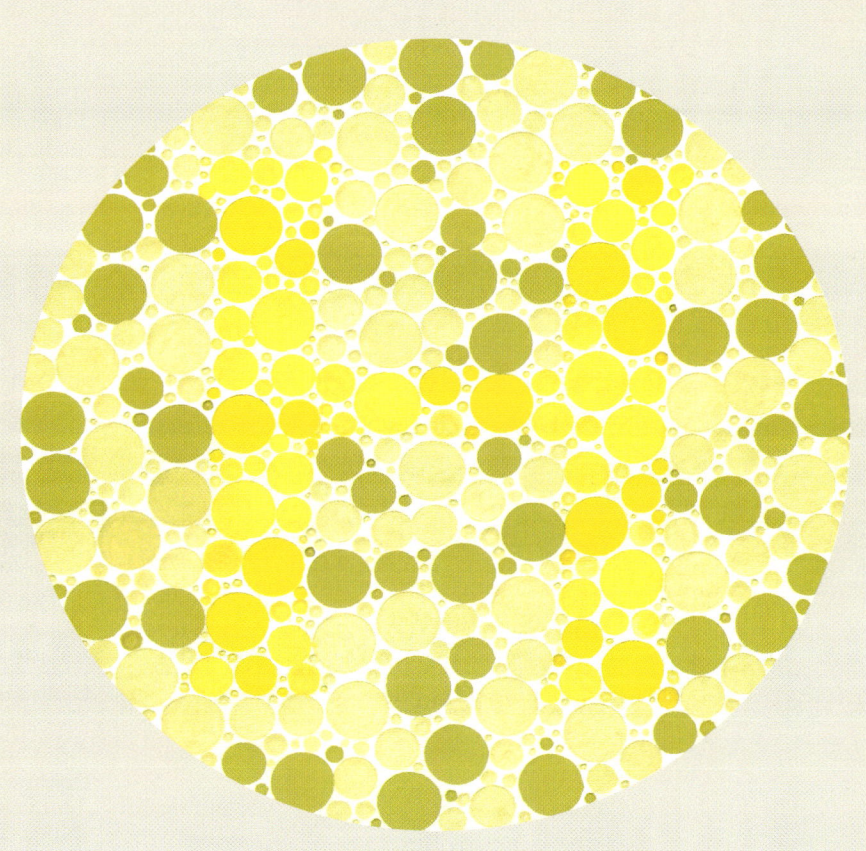

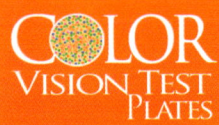

3. Animal figure group

Plate number	Normal	Color vision anomaly		Annotation
		Type	Result	
52	Swallow		Swallow	demonstration
53	Rabbit and duck	Red-green color vision anomaly	Duck	Distinguish red-green blindness and a part of weakness
54	Horse	Red-green color vision anomaly	Goat	Distinguish red-green blindness and a part of weakness
55	Cock	Red-green color vision anomaly	Can't read it	Distinguish red-green blindness
56	Goldfish	Red-green color vision anomaly	Can't read it	Distinguish red-green blindness
57	Bird	Red color vision anomaly	Can't read it	Distinguish red blindness
58	Horse	Red color vision anomaly	Can't read it	Distinguish red blindness and a part of red weakness
59	Swallow	Green color vision anomaly	Can't read it	Distinguish green blindness
60	Hen	Green color vision anomaly	Can't read it	Distinguish green blindness and a part of green weakness
61	Duck	Blue (violet) color vision anomaly	Can't read it	Distinguish blue (violet) blindness
62	Pigeon	Blue (violet) color vision anomaly	Can't read it	Distinguish blue (violet) blindness and a part of blue (violet) weakness
63	Deer	Yellow blindness	Can't read it	Distinguish yellow blindness

continued

Plate number	Normal	Color vision anomaly		Annotation
		Type	Result	
64	Butterfly	Strong degree of yellow weakness	Can't read it	Distinguish yellow weakness
65	Bull	Mild degree of yellow weakness	Can't read it	Distinguish yellow weakness
66	Elephant	Tiredness of color vision	Can read it at beginning, then deny it later	Distinguish the tiredness of color vision and latent color blindness
		Latent color blindness	Can't read it at beginning, then maybe can read it later	

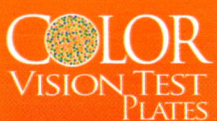

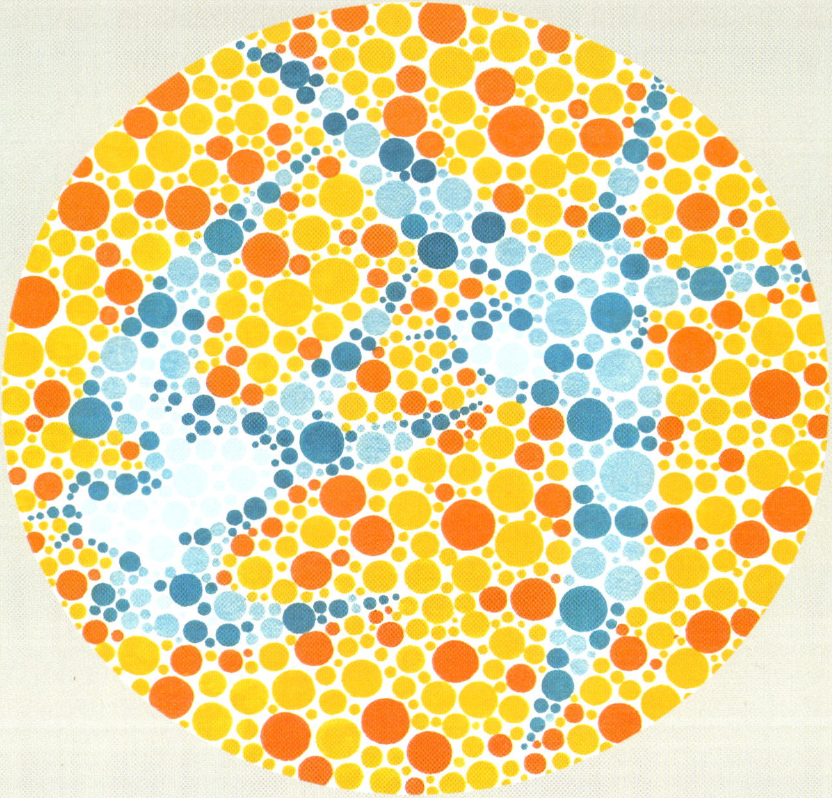

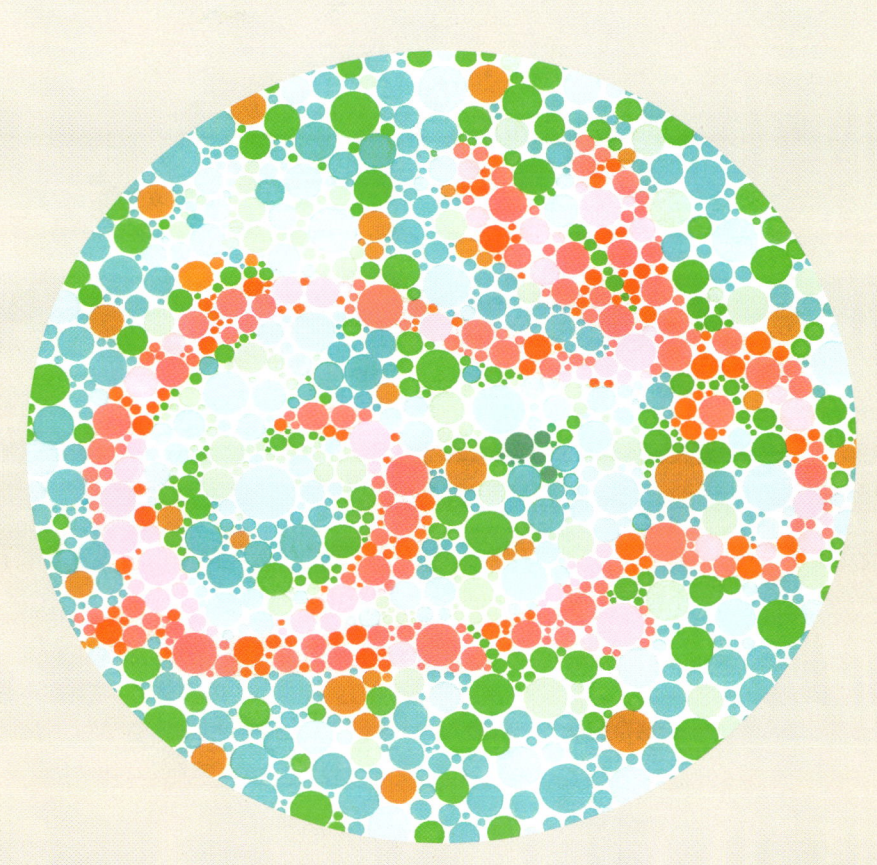

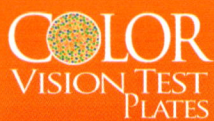

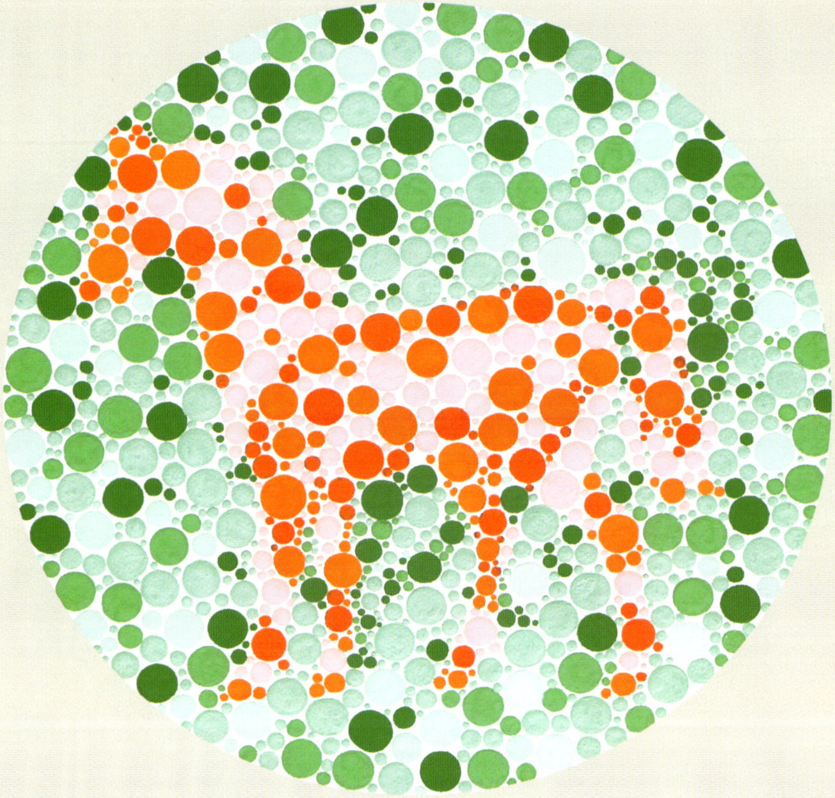

COLOR
VISION TEST
PLATES

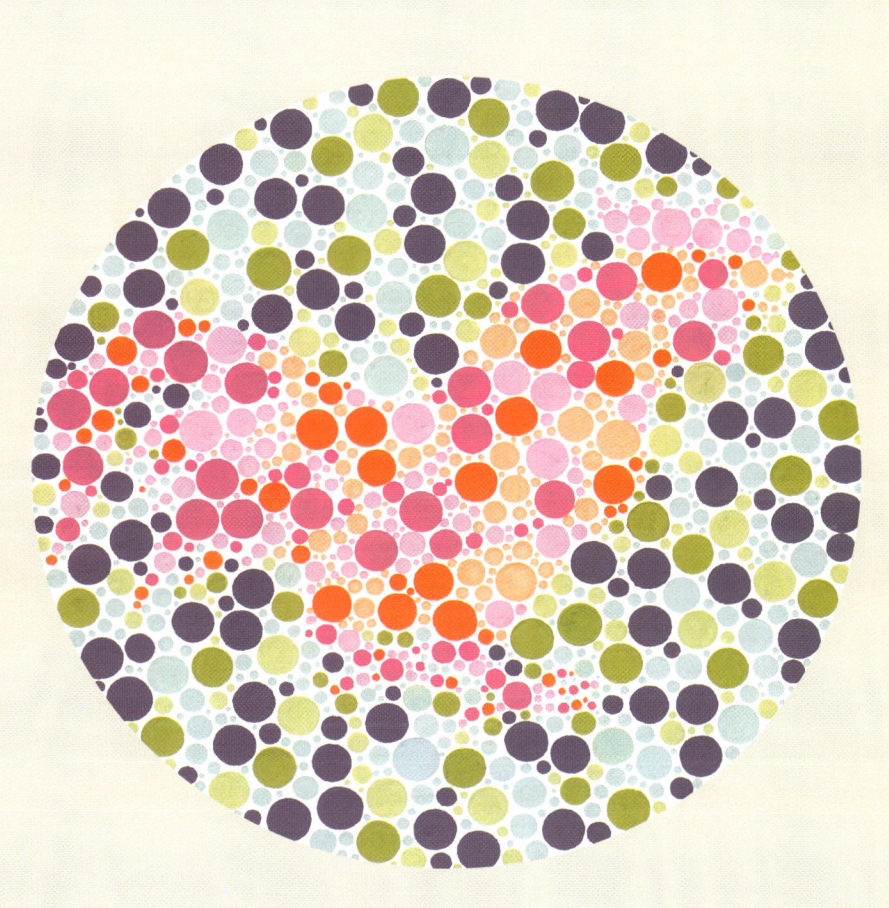

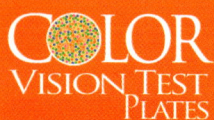

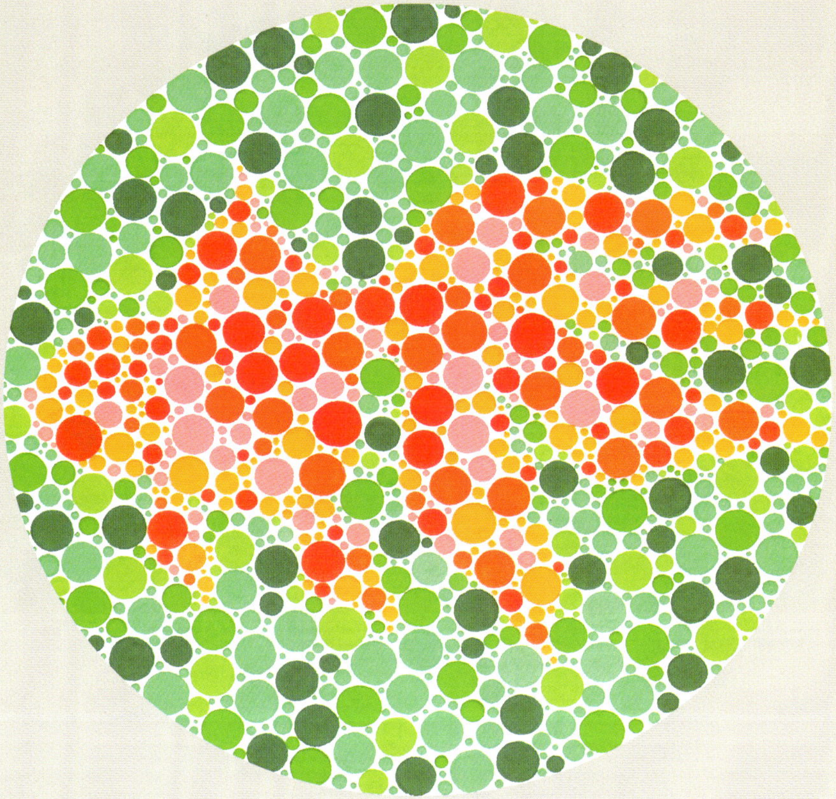

COLOR
VISION TEST
PLATES

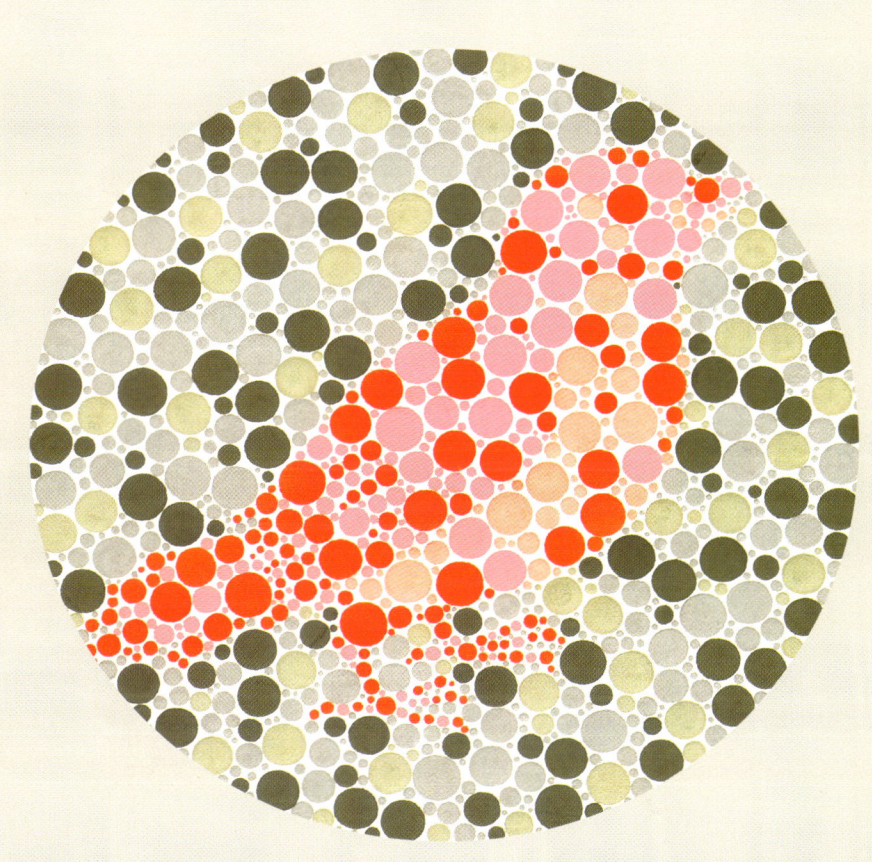

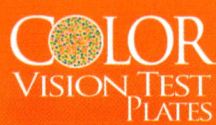

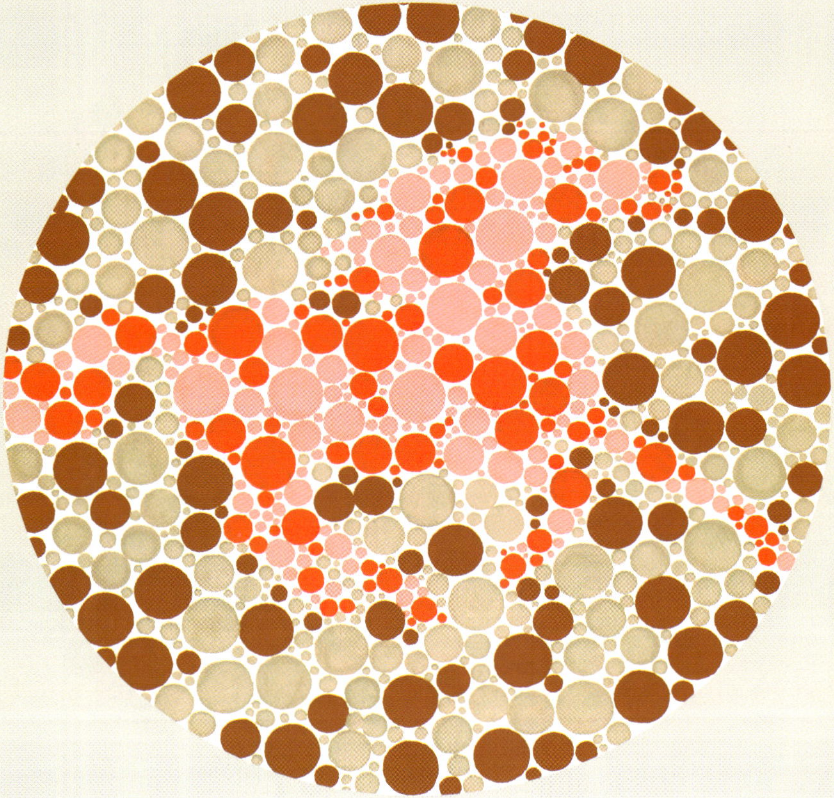

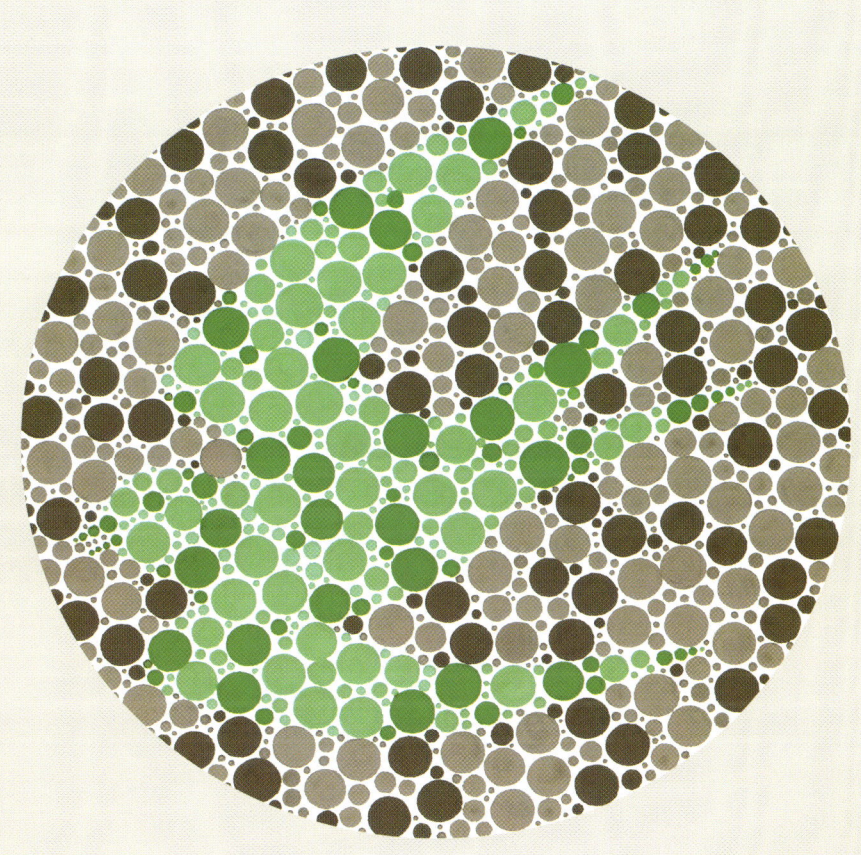

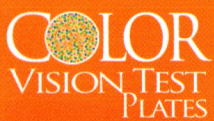

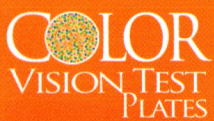

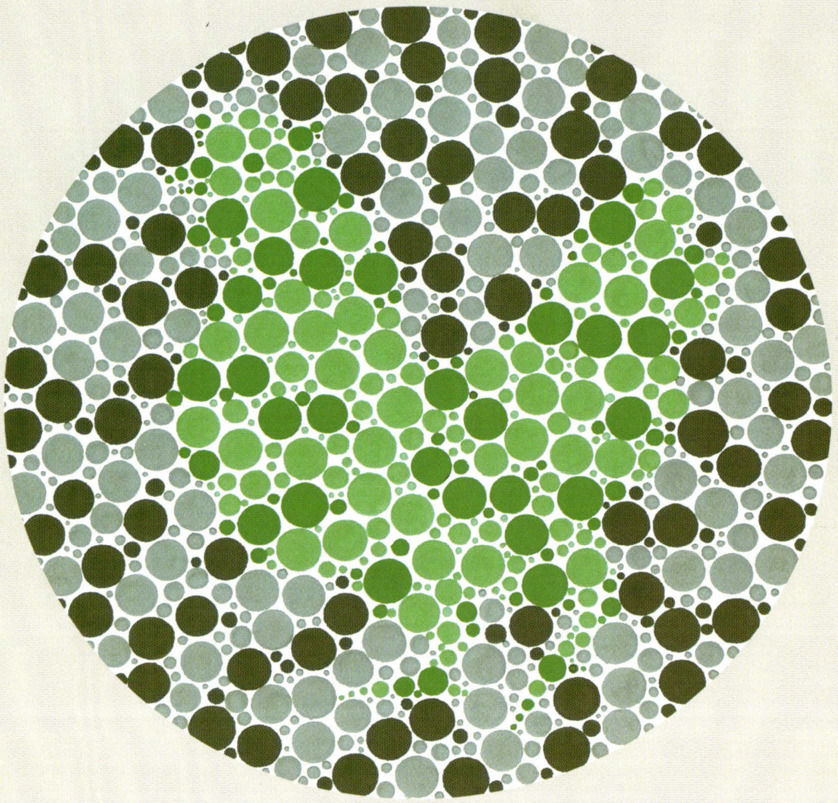

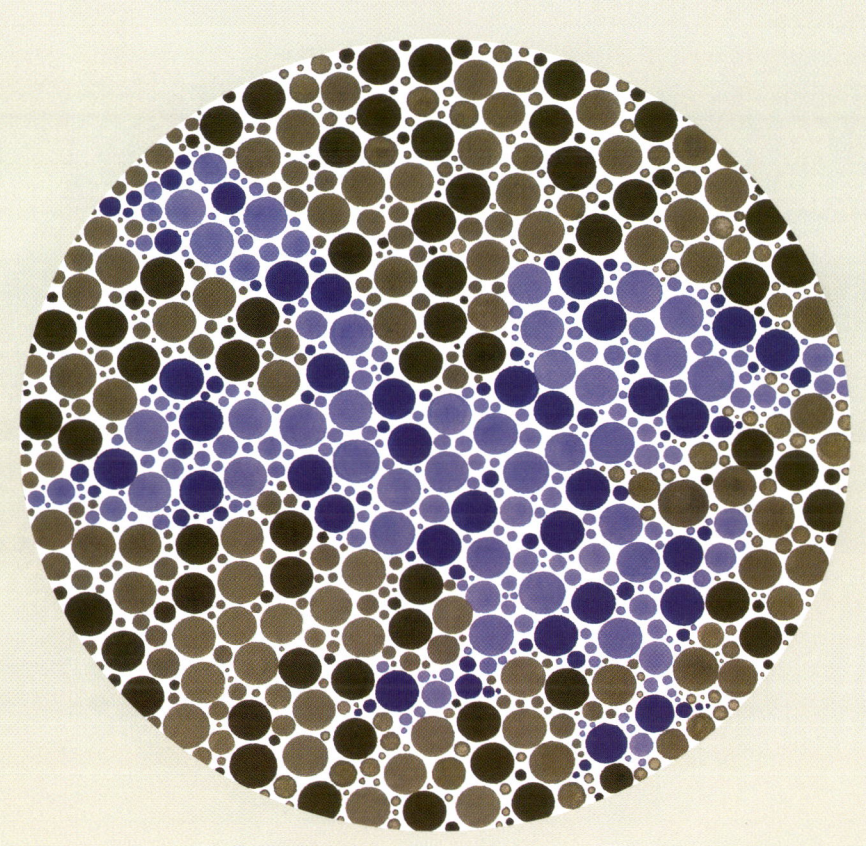

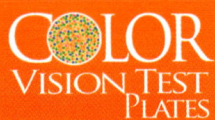

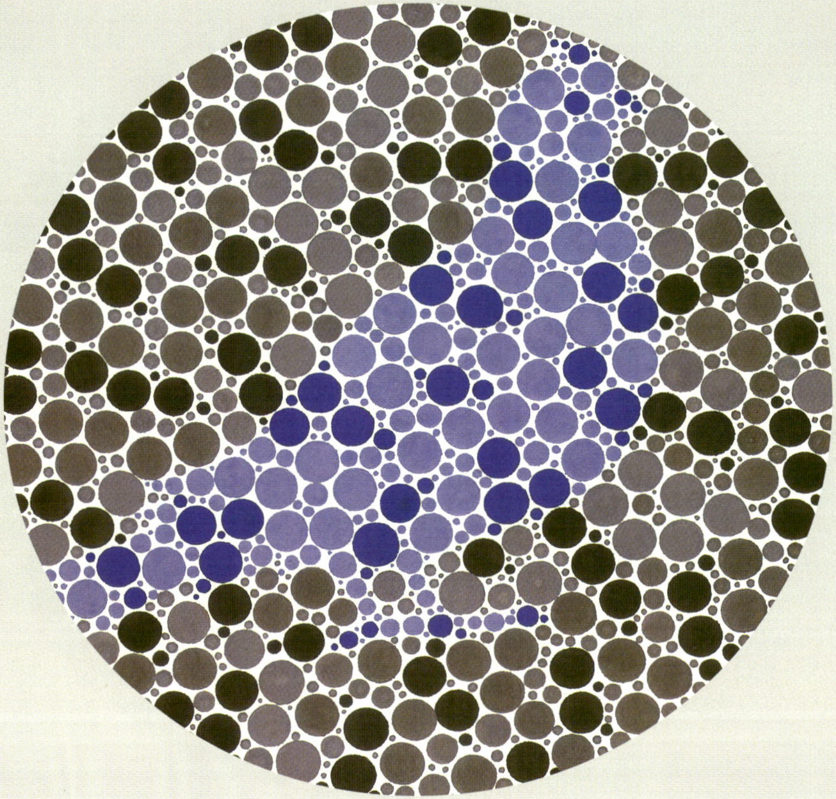

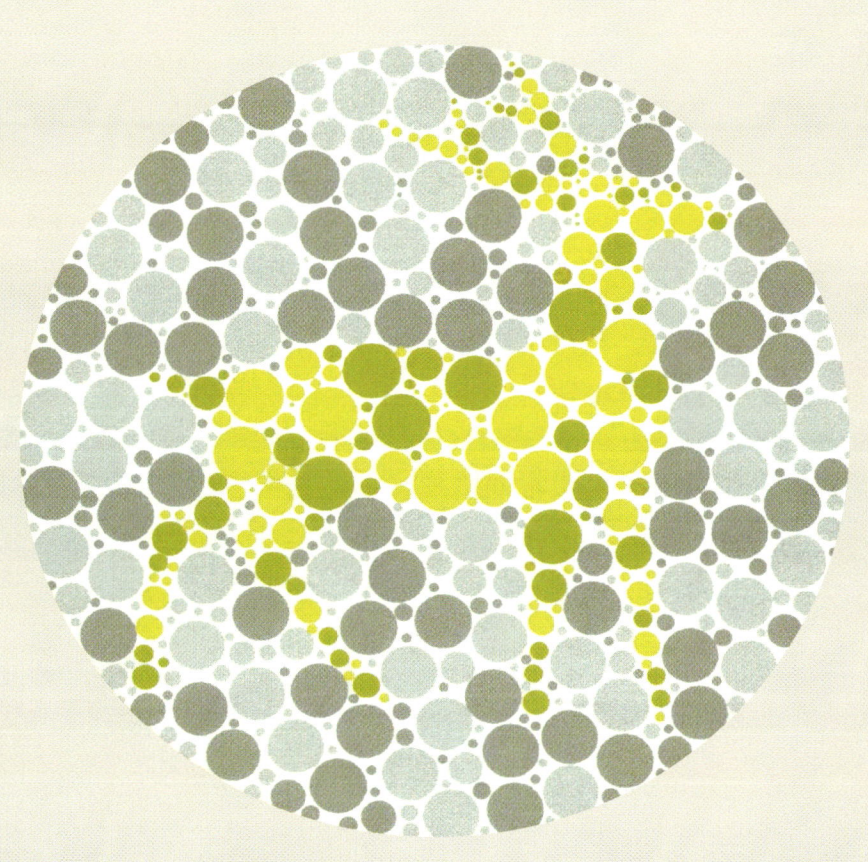

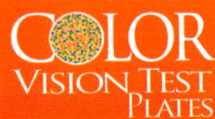

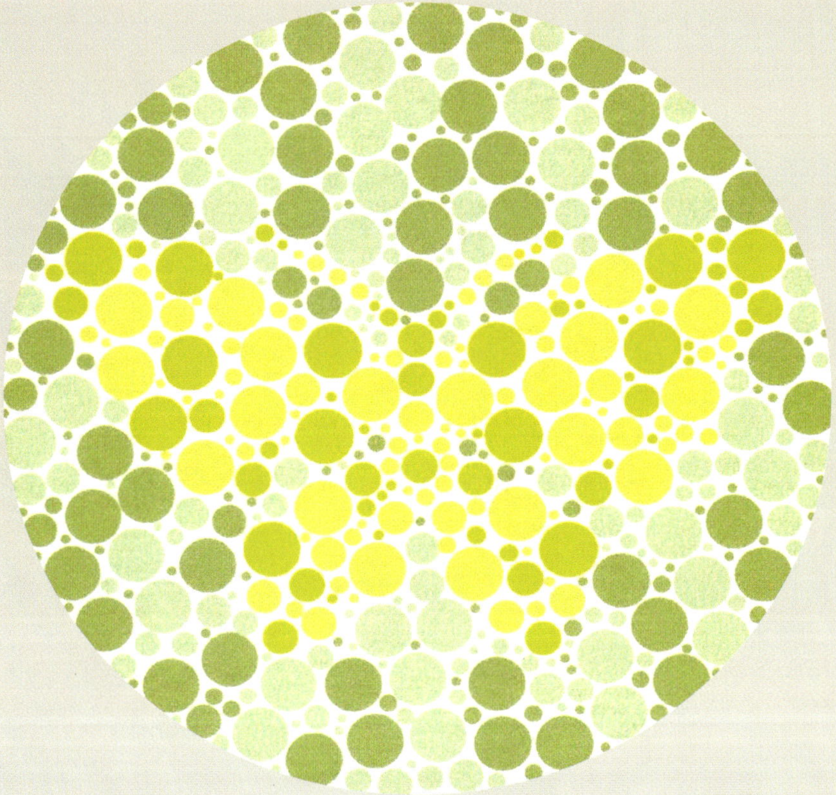

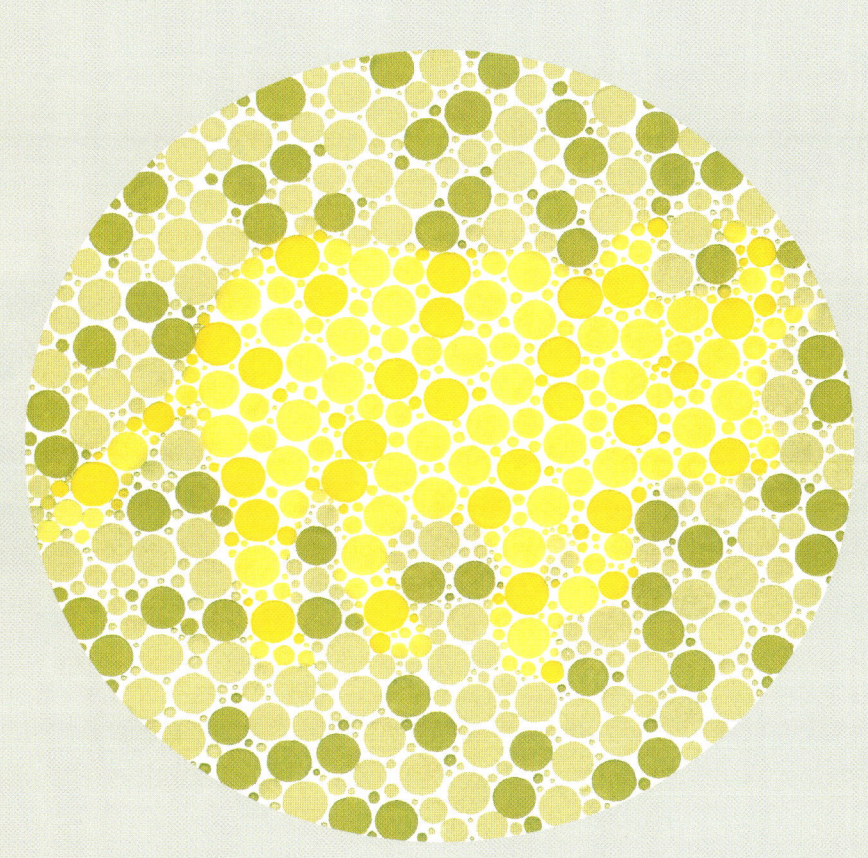

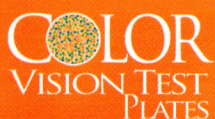

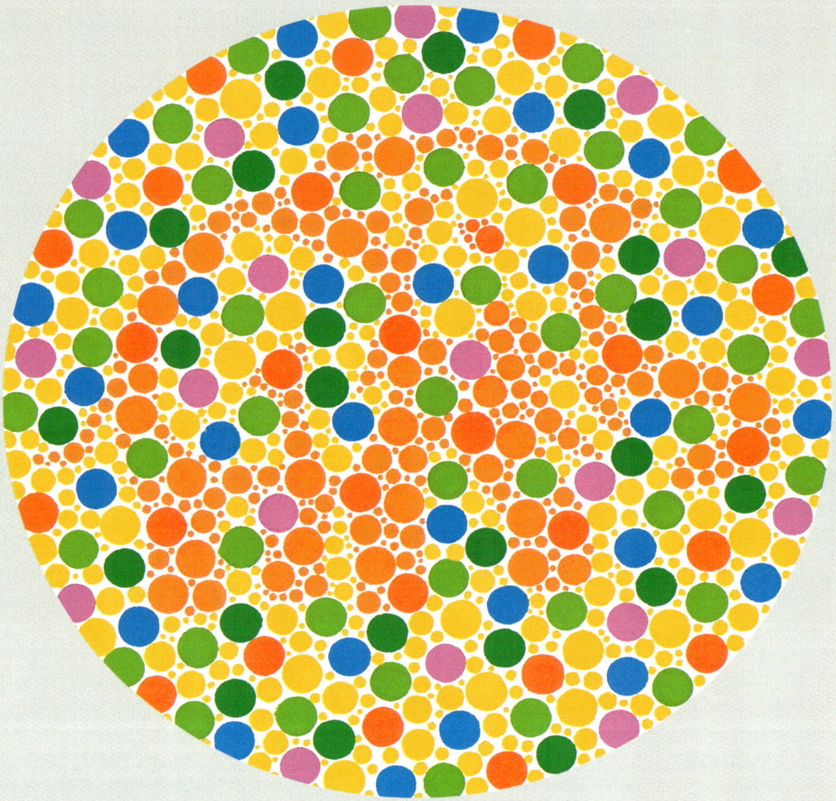

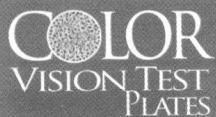

图书在版编目（CIP）数据

色觉检查图（英文）/ 王克长主编. 一北京：
人民卫生出版社，2008.3
ISBN 978−7−117−09176−3

Ⅰ．色... Ⅱ．王... Ⅲ．色觉试验−眼科检查−图谱
Ⅳ．R770.42−64

中国版本图书馆CIP数据核字（2007）第133282号

色觉检查图（英文）

主　　编：王克长
出版发行：人民卫生出版社（中继线 +8610-6761-6688）
地　　址：中国北京市丰台区方庄芳群园三区3号楼
邮　　编：100078
网　　址：http ://www. pmph. com
E - mail：pmph @ pmph. com
发　　行：zzg@pmph. com. cn
购书热线：+8610-6769-1034（电话及传真）
开　　本：889×1194　1/24
版　　次：2008 年 3 月第 1 版　2008 年 3 月第 1 版第 1 次印刷
标准书号：ISBN 978-7-117-09176-3／R・9177